MY HEALTH

MY PRIORITY

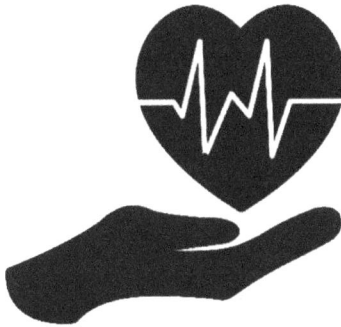

*Empowering Community
Health for our Pride*

MIRANDA NDIFON NZOYEM

Healthcare Professional and Educator

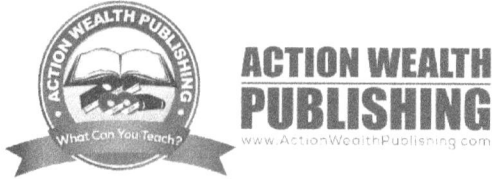

ACTION WEALTH PUBLISHING
www.ActionWealthPublishing.com

Kemp House
152-160 City Road
London, EC1V 2NX
United Kingdom

ISBN: 978-1-917451-07-9

Published by Miranda N. Nzoyem and Action Wealth Publishing
Printed and bound in the United Kingdom

To our dad, Pa Ndifon Daniel, and Mom, Ma Perpetua Ndifon, for their unwavering support throughout my life and for believing in education.

Given his tender age, I am also dedicating this book to our son, Vidal, Jr., for his resilience and the life lessons I am learning from him.

TABLE OF CONTENTS

ACKNOWLEDGEMENTS

I WOULD LIKE TO THANK my siblings for always standing by me and supporting me in being who I am today.

My colleagues for being a great team and my second family.

My family members and friends, who always believe in me.

My "husband" for the support we give each other.

My students for the role they play in my growth and development.

Also, thank you to the editor(s), manager, and the entire Action Wealth Publishing team for their support in carrying me through to the finish line of this project.

INTRODUCTION AND BACKGROUND

HEALTH IS A VITAL ASPECT of our lives, yet many communities face significant challenges in accessing the knowledge and resources necessary to maintain their well-being. As a healthcare professional with extensive experience, I have witnessed firsthand the health disparities that disproportionately affect the African or Black communities. This book, *My Health, My Priority: Empowering Community Health for Our Pride*, is born out of a deep desire to bridge these gaps, educate, and empower individuals to take control of their health, strengthening our collective well-being.

In this book, we will first delve into the unique health challenges African or Black communities face. Then, we will provide a comprehensive guide to understanding and managing common chronic diseases. More importantly, we will equip you with practical, actionable strategies for disease prevention and health maintenance, empowering you to take control of your health.

My primary purpose in authoring this book is to provide valuable health information to the African or Black population, focusing on common chronic diseases that are more prevalent within this community. This book is a collection of health advice and a tool to address the health disparities that disproportionately affect the Black community. By understanding these disparities and adopting the preventive measures and health maintenance strategies discussed in this book, we can work towards reducing the prevalence of these diseases and improving the overall health of our community.

Who Should Read This Book?

My Health, My Priority aims at the African or Black community, but its content is universal. Health challenges do not discriminate; everyone, regardless of their background, can find value in the preventive measures and health maintenance strategies discussed in this book. However, I have chosen to focus on the Black community due to the unique health challenges they face, the lack of targeted resources, and the need for increased awareness and education to decrease the prevalence of diseases.

Why Should You Trust My Insights?

I was born in Bamenda, in the Northwest region of Cameroon. Growing up, my life was shaped by the values of community and family, which were central to our way of living. My healthcare journey began when I moved to the

United States, facing numerous challenges in pursuing my education and establishing my career. Despite these obstacles, I remained committed to becoming a healthcare professional, driven by a passion for helping others and improving health outcomes within my community.

Through years of dedication and committed efforts, I earned my Master of Science in Nursing and became a nurse instructor. My experiences working with diverse populations and witnessing the recurring health issues among Black patients fueled my commitment to making a difference. This book culminates my experiences, education, and unwavering determination to provide the Black community with the tools and knowledge needed to achieve better health.

Why Are Health Disparities Still Affecting Our Community?

The Black community faces a higher prevalence of certain diseases compared to other populations. Conditions such as hypertension, heart failure, stroke, cancer, diabetes, asthma, and liver cirrhosis are more common and often more challenging to manage. Genetic, socio-economic, and cultural factors influence these health disparities. Studies have shown that the Black community frequently lacks access to resources and education about these specific health problems or health education in general (Baraka Muvuka, Ryan M. Combs, 2020).

This lack of information leads to delayed diagnoses, poor disease management, and worse health outcomes. By spreading awareness and providing practical guidance, I aim to empower individuals to make informed decisions, adopt healthier lifestyles, and reduce the incidence of these chronic diseases.

What Will You Achieve by Reading This Book?

Through *My Health, My Priority*, I aim to see readers make better life choices regarding their health. This book is designed to help readers:

* Understand common diseases prevalent in the Black community.

* Identify risk factors and unhealthy lifestyle habits contributing to these diseases.

* Adopt preventive measures and healthy habits to maintain good health.

* Assess family health history to anticipate and prevent potential health issues.

* Commit to improving your health and enhancing your overall quality of life, which includes increased longevity, better physical and mental well-being, cost savings, and a positive impact on personal and community relationships.

Health is like an eggshell fragile and precious. It is far better to safeguard it proactively than to regret neglecting it later. The adage "health is wealth" rings true; prioritizing disease prevention and health maintenance can save family resources and improve our overall quality of life. When we achieve better health individually, we contribute to the strength and prosperity of the entire Black community, fostering a sense of pride and unity.

Can You Take Charge of Your Health? *Yes! Of Course!*

By actively engaging with this information and implementing the healthy habits and choices outlined in this book, you can prevent chronic disease onset, manage existing health conditions more effectively, and improve your overall well-being. Look into your family health history, identify common issues, and proactively implement the preventive measures suggested here. By doing so, you will not only protect your health but also preserve your family resources from being depleted by long-term and costly medical treatments.

Prioritizing your health is not just a personal endeavor but an investment in the Black community health and pride. Healthy individuals make up a robust and vibrant community. When we care for ourselves, we set an example for others and uplift the community. Your role in this is crucial. Together, we can create a healthier, more informed, and empowered Black community, proud of its commitment to well-being.

In your pursuit of better health, remember that knowledge is power. With the information and strategies in this book, you can take charge of your health and make informed decisions that will benefit you and your loved ones. Let us embark on this path to better health together, prioritizing our well-being and creating a healthier, more informed community proud of its strength and resilience. Remember, while this book is aimed at the African or Black communities, its insights and strategies are universal and can benefit anyone seeking to improve their health.

Welcome to *My Health, My Priority*.

PROLOGUE I

THE QUIET CHILDHOOD

A QUIET CHILDHOOD can shape a person in profound and lasting ways, fostering introspection, observation, and a deep connection with one's inner world. Growing up in an environment marked by tranquility and reflection, children like me often find comfort in solitude or the close company of family and trusted friends. This upbringing nurtures a unique personal development, where imagination and self-reflection flourish without constant external stimulation.

Such a childhood cultivates a rich inner life characterized by empathy, creativity, and a heightened ability to observe and understand the world from a unique perspective. The quiet moments of these early years provide the space to explore thoughts, feelings, and dreams, leading to a keen sense of self-awareness and inner strength.

However, the path of a quiet child is not without its challenges. More reserved people may struggle to find their place or express themselves confidently in a world that often celebrates extroversion and social interaction. Sometimes, our quiet nature is misunderstood by peers and adults, who may mistake it for shyness or aloofness. Despite these challenges, a quiet childhood is incredibly enriching, fostering a deep appreciation for the simple things in life and laying a solid foundation for personal growth.

The qualities developed during these quiet moments patience, thoughtfulness, and resilience become invaluable as we navigate the complexities of adulthood with a calm and reflective approach. From this quiet, reflective foundation, my story begins, rooted in the experiences and lessons of my early years in Bamenda, Cameroon.

Growing up in Bamenda

Bamenda, nestled in the Northwest region of Cameroon, is more than just a geographical location; it is a place rich in culture, community, and traditions that profoundly shaped my early years. My childhood in Bamenda was marked by stability and a powerful sense of belonging. My parents raised me in the city where I was born, which became the backdrop for all my formative experiences. The town itself, with its lush landscapes and close-knit communities, fostered a unique upbringing where everyone knew each other, and the concept of community extended far beyond the immediate family.

A deep-rooted sense of community characterized life in Bamenda. My childhood was not confined to the walls of our home but extended into the streets and neighborhoods where I played with other children and interacted with numerous families. It was where distinctions between "my child" and "your child" blurred, as all the parents in the neighborhood looked out for each other's children. This collective upbringing instilled a sense of security and communal responsibility, values that have stayed with me throughout my life.

Religion plays a significant role in our daily lives. My Christian upbringing was deeply embedded in the fabric of our community, influencing our spiritual practices and social interactions. Sundays were reserved for church activities, where I participated in Sunday School and later joined the youth group. These activities were more than just religious obligations; they were opportunities for fellowship, learning, and personal growth. Through the church, I learned the importance of compassion, humility, and service values that became the cornerstone of my character.

However, one thing that always puzzled me was how often people would diagnose themselves with malaria whenever they felt unwell. Self-diagnosis was common in Bamenda, with many beginnings of treatment without proper medical advice or a true understanding of the various diseases that could present with similar symptoms.

Understanding the common diseases that disproportionately affect the Black population is crucial for communities like Bamenda to adopt healthier preventive measures and ensure the appropriate medical management of specific health issues. Improving health literacy and addressing cultural beliefs can promote better community health and help close the gaps in chronic health disparities.

In Bamenda, life was simple but rich with experiences that shaped my worldview. The stability of growing up in the same house, in the same town, and with the same people provided a consistent environment where I could develop a powerful sense of identity and belonging. Though seemingly uneventful to an outsider, my childhood was filled with the subtle yet profound experiences of communal living, cultural heritage, and spiritual growth that laid the foundation for the person I would become.

Shaping a Reserved Spirit

I was naturally reserved from an early age, a trait that set me apart in a community where outgoing personalities were more common. My quiet nature was not simply shyness but a deep-seated inclination towards introspection and observation. I often found myself on the fringes of social gatherings, not out of disinterest, but because I felt more comfortable in solitude or the company of a few close friends. This reserved nature shaped my early interactions, making me a keen listener and an observer of the world around me.

Growing up as a quiet child in Bamenda had its challenges. In a community where children were expected to be lively and vocal, my timidity was often misunderstood as aloofness or disinterest. I struggled to express myself, not because I lacked the words but because I was hesitant to share my thoughts and feelings openly. This internal struggle sometimes led to feelings of isolation as I watched others effortlessly engage in conversations and activities that I found daunting. However, my quietness also became a strength, allowing me to develop a rich inner life and a deep empathy for others.

My Christian upbringing played a crucial role in helping me navigate the challenges of being reserved. The church's teachings gave me a moral compass and a sense of purpose, even when I felt out of place among my peers. The values of humility, patience, and self-discipline, emphasized in Sunday School and other church activities, resonated with my natural disposition. Over time, I began to see my reserved nature not as a limitation but as a unique gift that allowed me to connect with others on a deeper level.

As I grew older, I realized that my quiet nature was not something to overcome but to embrace. It shaped how I interacted with the world, guiding me to channel my reservedness into thoughtful reflection and meaningful relationships. While I gradually became more outgoing, especially as I entered new phases of life, the core of my personality remained rooted in the quiet strength that had defined my childhood. This journey of self-acceptance was not always easy, but it was essential in helping me understand and appreciate the value of being true to myself.

I started finding my voice when I moved to the United States and began practicing nursing. As a healthcare provider, I learned the significance of advocating for patients and speaking on their behalf at vulnerable stages of their lives. This experience helped me begin to speak up more. Although I still prefer a quieter side of life, I have come to understand when it is necessary to raise my voice. Realizing I had much to contribute, I knew I could not remain as reserved as I had been. My passion for teaching also pushed me to step out of my comfort zone, knowing that effective communication was essential to achieving my goals.

Life's challenges further compelled me to find my voice, forcing me to stand up and speak out for myself, others in vulnerable situations, and the causes that truly matter to me. While I have progressed, people around me still often describe me as reserved and quiet. Being quiet is part of my nature, and I only push myself to speak up because I have learned the importance of communication, especially in healthcare. Authoring this book is an opportunity to add my voice to the conversation about the welfare and healthcare of the community, particularly the African community, which may need voices like mine to promote quality healthcare and a higher quality of life.

The Genesis of Lifelong Learning

My journey towards lifelong learning began early in my childhood, deeply influenced by my family and the educational opportunities available in Bamenda. Education was a core value in our household, and from an early age, I was encouraged to pursue knowledge with dedication and curiosity. My parents, who believed strongly in the transformative power of education, ensured that I attended school regularly and thoroughly engaged in academic activities. Their emphasis on learning was not merely about achieving academic success but cultivating a mindset of continuous growth and exploration.

In Bamenda, formal education was the primary path to personal and professional development. I attended local schools where dedicated teachers instilled in me the foundational reading, writing, and arithmetic skills. These early educational experiences sparked a curiosity that has stayed with me throughout my life. I was particularly drawn to subjects that allowed me to explore the world beyond my immediate surroundings, such as history and literature. These subjects opened my mind to innovative ideas and perspectives, fueling my desire to learn more and broadening my understanding of the world.

As I progressed through school, education became more than a requirement or a means to a future career—it became a passion. I began to engage in self-directed learning, eagerly seeking out books, articles, and other resources that piqued my interest. This shift towards independent learning allowed me to take control of my educational journey, exploring fascinating topics and deepening my knowledge in ways that extended beyond the traditional classroom setting.

The seeds of lifelong learning planted in my early years continued to grow as I moved through distinct phases of my life. Whether pursuing formal education or engaging in self-study, I remain committed to expanding my knowledge and skills. This commitment is not just about personal advancement but about becoming a more informed and capable individual who can contribute meaningfully to society. My early experiences in Bamenda taught me that learning is a lifelong process that requires dedication, curiosity, and a willingness to embrace innovative ideas.

Learning has always been a part of who I am. I have a deep love for acquiring knowledge, and I enjoy sharing what I have learned, especially when I believe it can make a difference in the world. Authoring this book, *My Health, My Priority*, is an extension of my learning process and a way to share the insights I have gained in disease prevention and health maintenance.

My educational journey began in Bamenda, where I completed my primary education. This led me to earn a Master of Science in Nursing as a Nurse Educator. My passion for formal and informal learning has been a constant in my life, and I look forward to continuing this journey of discovery and growth.

Challenges and Determination

Childhood is often a time of discovery, but for me, it was also a period marked by significant challenges that required determination and resilience. Growing up in Bamenda, I faced various obstacles that tested my resolve and shaped my character. Though not always dramatic, these challenges were formative, teaching me invaluable lessons about perseverance and the importance of self-motivation.

One of the primary challenges was balancing my natural reserve with the expectations of a communal society. As a quiet child, I often felt uncoordinated with the more extroverted children around me, leading to moments of self-doubt. I questioned whether I could truly fit in or express myself in a way others would understand and appreciate. However, rather than retreating further into myself, I began to push against these limitations, realizing that if I wanted to achieve my goals and be heard, I would need to step out of my comfort zone.

This realization led to a newfound determination. I started setting small, achievable goals to build confidence and expand my comfort zone. Whether participating more actively in class or taking on a leadership role in church, I consciously tried to challenge myself. Each success, no matter how small, reinforced my belief that I could overcome obstacles. This self-driven approach became a hallmark of my personality and would serve me well in the future.

As I grew older, this determination only strengthened. New challenges arose, particularly in my academic and professional pursuits, but the lessons I had learned in childhood remained with me. I understood that success was not always about natural talent or accessible opportunities; it was often about grit, persistence, and the willingness to keep pushing forward, even when the road was difficult. These early experiences taught me the value of resilience, an essential quality in my personal and professional life.

When I moved to the United States, the challenges I faced intensified. Until then, my parents had always provided for my needs, and I had never truly worked for myself. Suddenly, I found myself juggling work and school simultaneously a completely new experience that forced me to confront the realities of life. I attended school in the morning and worked in the afternoons or at night. Working night shifts was particularly challenging because I had never been a night person before moving to the U.S. Two weeks after arriving, I started the Certified Nursing Assistant program while searching for a job.

After completing the program, I secured employment and began attending college to complete the general education courses required for my nursing program. Balancing work and school was a significant challenge, but I stayed focused on becoming a registered nurse.

During my quest to become a nurse, I became pregnant with my son, adding another layer of complexity to my life. Now, I had to manage the demands of motherhood, school, and work simultaneously. It was incredibly challenging, but I remained focused on my goal. One thing that made it easier for me as a new mother and student was the support of my family, who were willing to help with my son whenever needed.

I gave birth in the middle of a semester and was back in class the following week, determined to continue my education. These experiences reinforced the lessons of resilience and determination that had been instilled in me since childhood, proving that no matter the challenges, I could overcome them by staying focused and persistent.

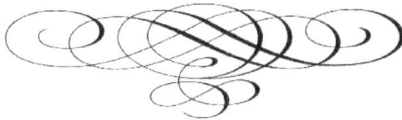

PROLOGUE II

BUILDING A LIFE OF PURPOSE AND BALANCE

BUILDING A LIFE OF PURPOSE and balance becomes increasingly crucial as childhood's quiet foundations transition into adulthood's complexities. This phase of life is marked by the pursuit of personal and professional goals, the nurturing of relationships, and the ongoing development of a keen sense of self. The lessons and values instilled during the early years are now put to the test, guiding decisions and actions as we navigate the intricate dance of balancing love, family, and ambition.

Balancing Love, Family, and Ambition

Balancing love, family, and ambition is a delicate and ongoing process that requires intentionality, resilience, and constant adjustment. As I transitioned into adulthood, these three elements became central to my life, each demanding time, energy, and focus. The challenge was managing these demands individually and harmonizing them so that each could thrive without compromising the others.

Love, in its various forms romantic, familial, and self-love is the foundation for a fulfilling life. For me, this meant nurturing my relationships with my husband, son, and extended family while ensuring that I maintained a healthy relationship with myself. Love provided the energy to pursue my ambitions and face the inevitable challenges. However, love alone was not enough; it needed to be balanced with pursuing personal and professional goals.

Family has always been a cornerstone of my life. The support and encouragement I received from my family played a critical role in my ability to pursue my ambitions. Managing family life, work, and being a student was far from easy, but having my family around, especially their willingness to assist my son, made a significant difference. There were times when the demands of my career clashed with my responsibilities at home, forcing me to make complex decisions. Navigating these moments taught me the importance of setting boundaries, seeking help when needed, and being adaptable to family life and work.

Ambition drove me to continue my education, advance my career, and strive for personal growth. My journey from a Certified Nursing Assistant to a Licensed Vocational Nurse and eventually to a Registered Nurse and Nurse Educator was fueled by an ardent desire to make a meaningful impact in my field. This ambition required long hours of study, late nights, and a commitment to continuous learning. Balancing this ambition with my family's needs and the desire to maintain a loving home environment was challenging but essential to achieving my goals.

One of the most challenging periods of my life was when I was pregnant, working, and studying simultaneously. Becoming a new mother while a student presented new challenges, but I remained focused on my dream of becoming a nurse. I attended school during the day and worked at night, often commuting long distances to complete my education. Despite the difficulties, I stayed committed to my purpose and, with God's help, completed my associate degree program with high honors. My Christian faith and natural spirit of calmness kept me focused and resilient amidst the challenges I faced. Because of my reserved nature, it was often difficult for others to tell when I was stressed, but I learned to navigate these trials gracefully.

Ultimately, I found that the key to balancing love, family, and ambition lies in remaining flexible and reassessing priorities as life evolves. It is about recognizing that there will be times when one area of life demands more attention than the others and being okay with that temporary shift in focus.

By staying true to my values and leaning on the support of those I love, I could pursue my ambitions without losing sight of what truly mattered. Even when faced with challenges, I never let them distract me from my goals and purpose I dreamed of becoming a nurse, caring for my son, and giving back to my community as much as possible. This journey taught me resilience, faith, and determination, the cornerstones of a balanced and fulfilling life.

Mentors and Role Models

Throughout my life, mentors and role models have played a pivotal role in shaping my perspectives, guiding my decisions, and inspiring me to strive for excellence. Through their actions and examples, these individuals have influenced how I approach my personal and professional life. While I have always been determined to carve my path, the insights and encouragement I received from these mentors and role models have been invaluable.

One of the most influential figures in my professional life has been my Assistant Nurse Manager, Alfonso. His steady and composed demeanor, even under pressure, taught me the importance of emotional intelligence in the workplace. I used to think of myself as calm and collected, but working with Alfonso made me realize the depth of steadfast composure.

His ability to maintain clarity and focus during stressful situations inspired me to develop my capacity for emotional resilience. This has been particularly important in nursing, where the stakes are high, and the ability to remain calm and make sound decisions is crucial.

Another key influence has been my manager, Arockiam, whose ambition and work ethic I deeply admire. She is a person who embodies determination and the relentless pursuit of excellence. Watching her navigate her career with purpose and intentionality has been a powerful reminder of the importance of setting high standards and pushing oneself to achieve them. Her example has encouraged me to maintain a similar drive and ambition in my career, always striving to reach new heights.

Beyond the workplace, my personal life has been enriched by the influence of family and friends who have served as role models. A close friend who is a medical doctor, Dr. Fombi, has inspired me with his simplicity, open-mindedness, and easygoing nature. His approach to life has taught me to remain grounded, to value the simple things, and to maintain an open heart and mind. His influence has helped me see life from different perspectives, reminding me of the importance of humility and diverse viewpoints.

My parents have also been lifelong role models, instilling in me the values of love, generosity, and kindness. Growing up, I watched them extend these values to everyone around them, treating each person with respect and compassion. Their actions taught me the importance of giving back to the community and living a life rooted in serving others. These lessons have stayed with me, guiding how I interact with others and influencing my desire to contribute meaningfully to my community.

Lastly, my son has become a source of inspiration in my life. His optimistic view of the world and his belief in the goodness of people have encouraged me to adopt a more positive outlook. He constantly reminds me that the world is filled with potential and beauty despite our challenges. His youthful enthusiasm and unyielding belief in good have made me strive to see the world through his eyes with hope and positivity.

In summary, my mentors and role models have given me invaluable lessons and examples. They have helped me navigate the complexities of life and work, offering guidance, inspiration, and support when I needed it most. While I am committed to forging my path, I recognize that the influence of these individuals has been instrumental in shaping who I am today. Their impact on my life reminds me of the importance of surrounding oneself with people who inspire, challenge, and support you in your journey toward personal and professional growth.

Foundational Principles and Faith

Foundational principles and faith have been the bedrock of my life, guiding my decisions, actions, and interactions with others. These core values, deeply rooted in my Christian upbringing and reinforced throughout my life, have given me a sense of purpose and direction, especially during challenging times. They are the compass by which I navigate the complexities of life, helping me to remain grounded and focused on what truly matters.

I was taught the importance of integrity, humility, and compassion early on. These principles were not just abstract concepts but were demonstrated daily by my parents and community. Integrity meant doing the right thing, even when no one was watching. It meant being honest in my dealings with others and staying true to my word. This value has been essential in my personal and professional life, particularly in nursing, where trust and reliability are paramount. Upholding integrity in all aspects of my life has earned me the respect of colleagues, patients, and loved ones, and it continues to guide my actions.

Humility is another principle that has shaped my worldview. I have always believed in acknowledging that there is always more to learn and that others have valuable insights and experiences. This humility has allowed me to approach each new situation with an open mind and a willingness to listen and learn from others. It has also helped me remain approachable and empathetic, traits crucial to my professional nurse role and relationships. Humility reminds me that success is not solely a product of my efforts but also the result of the support and guidance of those around me.

Compassion has been a guiding force in my interactions with others. Growing up, I witnessed my parents' unwavering commitment to helping those in need, whether offering a helping hand to a neighbor or supporting someone going through a tough time. This instilled a profound responsibility to care for others, a principle central to my nursing career. Compassion drives me to provide my patients with the best care possible and approach each person I encounter with kindness and understanding.

My Christian faith has been the cornerstone that ties all these principles together. It has provided me with a framework for understanding the world and my place within it. My faith teaches me to love others as I love myself, to forgive, and to serve selflessly. It has given me the strength to persevere through life's challenges, knowing that my struggles have a greater purpose. In times of uncertainty or difficulty, my faith has been a source of comfort and resilience, reminding me that I am never alone and can always find hope in God's plan.

Central to my faith is the belief in the power of knowledge, as the Bible emphasizes the importance of acquiring and sharing it. "My people perish for lack of knowledge," a biblical verse that resonates deeply with me, highlights knowledge's critical role in overcoming life's challenges, including health-related ones. This belief has fueled my passion for health literacy, particularly in addressing the health disparities that disproportionately affect the Black community.

I see knowledge as a powerful tool that empowers individuals to take control of their health and well-being. My desire to become an author stems from this understanding— by sharing knowledge through educational resources and awareness campaigns, mainly targeting the Black community, we can close the gaps in health disparities and promote better health outcomes.

Combining these foundational principles and my faith has shaped the person I am today. They have influenced how I approach my work, relationships, and goals. Whether it is making a difficult decision, supporting a loved one, or facing a personal challenge, these values guide me every step of the way. They remind me to stay true to myself, treat others with respect and compassion, and trust in the path laid out for me.

As I continue living, the above principles and my faith remain constant, providing me with the clarity and strength to navigate life's difficulties. They are values I strive to live by and the essence of my identity. Through them, I have found a sense of purpose beyond personal achievement, rooted in service, love, and a commitment to improving the world.

From CNA to RN

Upgrading from a Certified Nursing Assistant (CNA) to a Registered Nurse (RN) was one of the most challenging yet rewarding paths I have ever embarked on. My nursing career has been a series of small, deliberate steps, each building on the last and each bringing me closer to my goal. Starting as a CNA, I gained valuable hands-on patient care experience while taking general education (GE) courses as prerequisites for admission into a registered nursing program. My goal was clear: to enter a registered nursing program, but the path was far from straightforward.

While working as a CNA, I was fortunate to gain admission into the Licensed Vocational Nursing (LVN) program, a step I took despite my challenging circumstances. My faith and determination kept me focused on my dream of becoming a Registered Nurse. I knew that each program, each course, and each shift was a building block toward that goal. Even though I initially aimed for a generic nursing program, I seized the opportunity to start the LVN program, which was closer to home. I could begin this journey while awaiting admission into a Registered Nursing Program. By God's grace, I completed the LVN program after two years, which brought me one step closer to achieving my dream.

Upon graduating from the LVN program, I did not hesitate to seize the next opportunity. I gained admission into an LVN to RN program, even though it required a significant commute. The distance and the challenges were daunting, but I was ready for the challenge. Within a year, I completed the program, sat for the RN board exams, and obtained my RN license. This monumental achievement culminated years of hard work, sacrifice, and unwavering commitment to my goals.

I did not stop there. After working as an RN for two years, I pursued further education by enrolling in a Bachelor of Science in Nursing (BSN) program. Following a brief break, I continued my education by entering a Master of Science in Nursing (MSN) program. Each step in my educational journey was driven by my desire to gain more knowledge and expertise in nursing, especially given that our world is changing rapidly. I look forward to acquiring even more knowledge in nursing practice as I continue to grow professionally.

The progression from CNA to RN and beyond was not just about career advancement; it was a transformative experience that shaped my identity as a healthcare professional. It required resilience, adaptability, and a deep commitment to my goals. This journey reinforced my belief that overcoming challenges and achieving one's dreams with faith, determination, and proper support is possible.

As I reflect, I realize that each step, no matter how small, was crucial in building the foundation for the nurse I am today. My experiences have taught me that success is not achieved overnight but through consistent effort, learning, and growing. This understanding drives me to continue seeking knowledge and improving my practice, knowing that every new skill and piece of knowledge I acquire makes me a better nurse and allows me to provide the best care possible to my patients.

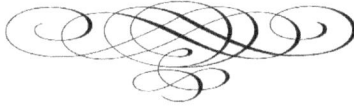

PART ONE

UNDERSTANDING HEALTH DISPARITIES

CHAPTER ONE

THE STATE OF BLACK HEALTH

"Black health is shaped by more than just statistics—our experiences, challenges, and resilience define it. True health equity begins when we address all of these."

Overview of Health Disparities Between Black and Other Populations.

HEALTH DISPARITIES BETWEEN Black population and other racial and ethnic groups have long been a critical issue in public health. These disparities refer to the differences in how various groups of people are affected by healthcare practices or disease processes. Throughout my nursing education, I have learned extensively about these disparities, particularly how Black communities are disproportionately affected by certain diseases compared to other races, such as the white population.

Historically, Black population or Africans have faced significant barriers to accessing quality healthcare, resulting in poorer health outcomes. These disparities manifest in numerous ways, including higher rates of chronic diseases such as hypertension, diabetes, and cardiovascular diseases. For instance, Black adults are more likely to suffer from hypertension at earlier ages and with greater severity, leading to higher rates of heart disease and stroke. Similarly, the prevalence of diabetes is significantly higher among Black individuals, contributing to a more significant burden of complications such as kidney failure, amputations, and vision loss.

Cancer outcomes also highlight the stark disparities between Black population and other groups. Black men have the highest rates of prostate cancer and are more likely to die from the disease than men of different races. Similarly, Black women are more likely to die from breast cancer despite having lower incidence rates as compare to their white counterparts. These disparities in cancer outcomes are often attributed to later-stage diagnoses, lower access to screening and preventive services, and differences in treatment received.

Maternal and infant health is another area where disparities are pronounced. Black women are three to four times more likely to die from pregnancy-related complications than white women, and Black infants have significantly higher mortality rates than infants of other races. These disparities are often linked to a combination of factors, including lack of access to quality prenatal care, higher rates of chronic conditions such as hypertension and diabetes that are likely to get worse during pregnancy, and systemic issues like racism and bias in healthcare.

Mental health is yet another domain where Black population face significant disparities. Black individuals are less likely to receive mental health services compared to white individuals, and when they do, the quality of care is often lower. The stigma surrounding mental health within Black communities, combined with a lack of culturally competent care, exacerbates these disparities. As a result, mental health conditions such as depression, anxiety, and PTSD often go untreated, leading to worse outcomes.

The COVID-19 pandemic has further exposed and exacerbated these health disparities. Black populations have experienced disproportionately higher rates of COVID-19 infections, hospitalizations, and deaths compared to other groups. This disparity is due to factors such as higher rates of underlying health conditions, limited access to healthcare, and the disproportionate impact of social determinants of health, such as income inequality, housing instability, and employment in essential but high-risk jobs.

Social determinants of health—such as economic stability, education, neighborhood and physical environment, and access to healthcare—play a significant role in perpetuating health disparities among Black populations. For example, lower socioeconomic status is associated with limited access to nutritious and healthy food, safe environments for physical activity, and quality healthcare services. These conditions contribute to the higher prevalence of chronic diseases and poorer overall health outcomes among blacks.

Cultural factors also influence health disparities. Mistrust of the healthcare system, rooted in historical abuses such as the Tuskegee Syphilis Study, continues to impact Black individuals' willingness to seek care. This mistrust, combined with experiences of discrimination and bias in healthcare settings, can lead to delays in seeking treatment, lower adherence to medical advice, and worse health outcomes.

Studies have consistently shown that Black people are disproportionately affected by chronic health conditions compared to other races. According to Ronald L. S. and Man-Kit L., among others, Black populations are more likely to suffer from these chronic conditions, which contribute to the widening gap in health disparities. Addressing these disparities requires a multifaceted approach that includes improving access to quality healthcare, addressing social determinants of health, increasing health literacy, and promoting culturally competent care.

In this book, *My Health, My Priority*, my goal is to identify these common health issues and propose possible healthy lifestyles or practical solutions for disease prevention and health maintenance to improve the quality of life in the Black community. The objective is to create opportunities to assist the African community in improving health outcomes and closing the gaps in healthcare disparities. By focusing on the chronic health disorders that significantly affect the African community, we can work towards closing these gaps and achieving better health for all.

In conclusion, health disparities between Black population and other racial and ethnic groups result from a complex interplay of factors. Understanding these disparities is the first step toward addressing them and ensuring that all individuals, regardless of race, can achieve their best health. As we progress in this discussion, we must recognize the urgency of addressing these disparities and commit to actions that will improve health outcomes for the Black community.

Statistical Data Highlighting the Prevalence of Certain Diseases Among Blacks.

Understanding the health disparities faced by Black population requires examining statistical data that highlights the prevalence of certain diseases within these communities. This data is crucial not only for illustrating the scope of the problem but also for guiding efforts to address these disparities and improve health outcomes.

Throughout my nursing career, I have gained valuable knowledge and made critical observations about how Black people are disproportionately affected by chronic health issues such as hypertension, heart failure, stroke, diabetes, and obesity. These observations are backed by numerous studies, confirming the extent of these disparities.

Hypertension, often referred to as the "silent killer," is more prevalent among Black adults, with nearly 57% affected compared to about 43% of their white counterparts, (Centers for Disease Control and Prevention, CDC). This condition can lead to severe complications such as heart disease, stroke, and kidney failure. Studies also show that the management of high blood pressure is better among whites than Black people, with 50.8% of whites achieving better control compared to 44.6% of Black people. This disparity highlights the need for targeted interventions to improve blood pressure management among Africans.

Diabetes is another chronic condition that disproportionately affects Black population. The American Diabetes Association reports that 12.7% of Black adults have diabetes, compared to 7.4% of white adults. According to Wendy L., Kimberly A. C., Rosemarie D., et al., the prevalence of Type 2 diabetes mellitus is 13.2% in Black people, compared to 12.8% in Hispanics and 7.6% in whites.

This increased risk is influenced by factors such as obesity, physical inactivity, and dietary habits prevalent in many Black communities due to socio-economic challenges. The consequences of poorly managed diabetes include heart disease, kidney disease, and nerve damage, making it a significant public health concern.

Obesity rates are also alarmingly high in Black communities, contributing to the higher prevalence of associated chronic conditions. The U.S. Department of Health and Human Services reports that 75.7% of Black people are obese compared to 71.6% of whites. Similarly, Wendy L. et al. found that 38.4% of Black people are obese, compared to 32.6% of Hispanics and 28.6% of whites. Obesity is a significant risk factor for conditions such as diabetes, heart disease, and stroke, which are already disproportionately affecting Black populations.

Cardiovascular diseases, including heart disease and stroke, are the leading causes of death among Black people. Although the prevalence of heart disease is slightly lower among Black people (5.2%) compared to Whites (5.6%), the death rate from heart disease is significantly higher in the Black community. According to the U.S. Department of Health and Human Services, 208.6 deaths per 100,000 occur in the Black population due to heart disease, compared to 166.4 deaths per 100,000 in whites. The gender-specific death rate is also higher in Black people, with 267.5 deaths per 100,000 Black men compared to 210.7 deaths per

100,000 white men and 165.0 deaths per 100,000 Black women compared to 129.6 deaths per 100,000 white women.

Renal failure is another condition where disparities are evident. Studies show that Black children are less likely to receive a kidney transplant than their white counterparts, with only 16.3% of Black children receiving a transplant compared to 41.8% of white children. This stark difference in healthcare management highlights the systemic inequities that Black populations face in receiving life-saving treatments.

Cancer statistics reveal similarly troubling disparities. Black men have the highest incidence and mortality rates for prostate cancer, with a 76% higher risk of death from the disease compared to white men. Black women, although less likely to be diagnosed with breast cancer than white women, are 40% more likely to die from it. These disparities are primarily due to differences in access to screening, early detection, treatment, and socio-economic factors affecting overall health.

The COVID-19 pandemic has further exposed and exacerbated these health disparities. Black Americans have been disproportionately affected by the virus, with higher rates of infection, hospitalization, and death compared to other racial and ethnic groups. The CDC reports that Black Americans are nearly three times more likely to die from COVID-19 than white Americans, a disparity driven by pre-existing health conditions, limited access to healthcare, and socio-economic challenges that increase exposure to the virus.

Mental health is another area where significant disparities exist. Black adults are more likely to experience severe psychological distress than white adults, yet they are less likely to receive treatment. When they do seek help, the care they receive is often of lower quality. The under-treatment of mental health conditions in the Black community exacerbates other health issues and contributes to the overall health disparities experienced by this population.

These statistical data points highlight the urgent need for focused and culturally competent public health interventions aimed at reducing the prevalence of these diseases and improving health outcomes in Black communities. The high death rate in the Black community can be reduced with health literacy and adequate healthcare resources. Inadequate access to healthcare, coupled with a lack of resources and targeted information, contribute to these disparities.

Conclusively, health disparities between Black populations and other racial and ethnic groups result from a complex interplay of factors. Understanding these disparities is crucial for ensuring everyone can achieve their best health regardless of race. By educating ourselves and others, we can take meaningful steps toward creating a healthier and more equitable society where everyone can attain the best possible health.

Socio-Economic and Cultural Factors Contribute to These Disparities

Health disparities in the Black community result from a complex mix of socio-economic and cultural factors. These factors contribute directly to unequal health outcomes, leading to higher rates of chronic diseases, lower life expectancy, and worse overall health in Black population compared to their white counterparts. Recognizing how these disparities manifest helps us understand the gaps in healthcare delivery and outcomes within the Black community.

The Impact of Socio-Economic Factors on Health Outcomes

Socio-economic factors, including income, employment, education, and housing, play a significant role in shaping health outcomes for Black individuals. For example, low-income Black families often have reduced access to essential healthcare services, leading to delayed diagnoses and limited access to treatment. This delay results in worsened outcomes for conditions such as hypertension, diabetes, and heart disease, which disproportionately affect Black populations.

The U.S. Census Bureau reports that 19.5% of Black Americans live below the poverty line, compared to only 8.2% of whites (U.S. Census Bureau, 2020). This economic disparity worsens health outcomes as families struggle to afford nutritious food, secure housing, and regular medical care. Moreover, stable employment with health benefits remains elusive for many Black Americans or Africans, further limiting access to preventive care and necessary treatments.

Educational Disparities and Health Outcomes

The link between education and health outcomes is well-established, with lower educational attainment often resulting in reduced health literacy and poorer overall health. According to the National Center for Education Statistics, only 25% of Black adults have a bachelor's degree or higher, compared to 40% of white adults. This educational gap perpetuates health disparities, as individuals with lower education levels may lack the knowledge to manage chronic diseases, access healthcare resources, or understand the importance of regular medical visits.

In the Black community, limited access to higher education, underfunded schools, and systemic barriers to academic advancement all contribute to worse health outcomes. Poor health literacy, a direct result of these educational challenges, often leads to higher rates of preventable diseases, like hypertension and diabetes, which could be better managed or avoided with timely intervention.

Environmental Factors and Health Risks

Environmental factors also exacerbate health disparities. Black communities often have limited access to grocery stores that sell fresh produce, clean parks for exercise, and healthcare facilities. This lack of resources increases the risk of chronic conditions such as obesity and diabetes. Moreover, Black neighborhoods frequently face exposure to environmental toxins, such as pollution, which leads to a higher incidence of respiratory illnesses such as asthma and other chronic diseases.

The Cultural Lens of Health Disparities

Cultural factors, including traditional beliefs and practices, further contribute to health disparities. For example, in many African communities, being overweight is often viewed as a sign of wealth and well-being, whereas in Western societies, it is associated with poor health. These cultural perceptions can lead to higher rates of obesity, which in turn increases the risk for lifelong diseases such as diabetes, hypertension, and cardiovascular diseases.

The cultural stigma around mental health also plays a critical role. Black communities often view mental health issues as a sign of weakness, which discourages individuals from seeking help. Untreated mental health conditions, such as depression or anxiety, can worsen physical health, further increasing the burden of chronic diseases.

While it is essential to recognize the various socio-economic and cultural factors contributing to health disparities in the Black community, the root causes behind these disparities—such as systemic barriers, racism, and inequitable access to healthcare—will be explored further in Chapter Two. For now, it is crucial to understand how these disparities manifest in everyday life, shaping the health outcomes of Black individuals and communities.

The Role of Healthcare Access and Systemic Barriers in Perpetuating Health Disparities.

As a healthcare provider, I understand the critical importance of access to healthcare for managing chronic conditions like heart failure, diabetes, kidney failure, and hypertension. Often, patients with these chronic health conditions are readmitted to the hospital quite often due to a lack of prescription refills, no access to medications, or limited access to primary care doctors. Many of these chronic conditions require daily medicines for health maintenance. While prevention is critical for those at high risk, once a person is diagnosed, access to healthcare becomes imperative, regardless of lifestyle management.

For instance, a patient with kidney failure who is on dialysis will need weekly healthcare access, and a patient recovering from a stroke may need access to rehabilitation services. Given that Black people are disproportionately affected by these chronic health conditions compared to other races, access to healthcare is a significant factor for the Black community to managing these lifelong diseases. It is also noted that race plays a vital role in health disparities, with being Black often placing one at a disadvantage in accessing healthcare (Ronald L. S., Man-Kit L., et al.).

Access to healthcare is a fundamental right and a critical determinant of health. However, for many Black people, access to quality healthcare remains a significant challenge, perpetuating health disparities and contributing to poorer health outcomes. Systemic barriers within the healthcare system further exacerbate these disparities, creating a cycle of inequity that is difficult to break. Understanding and addressing these barriers is essential for ensuring that all individuals can achieve optimal health.

Geographic Barriers and Healthcare Deserts

One of the most significant barriers to healthcare access is the geographic location of healthcare facilities. Many Black communities, particularly those in rural or economically disadvantaged urban areas, are situated in healthcare deserts—areas with limited access to hospitals, clinics, and primary care providers. In these regions, the nearest healthcare facility may be miles away, making it difficult for residents to receive timely care. This lack of proximity to healthcare services often leads to delayed diagnoses, untreated conditions, and a reliance on emergency care, all of which contribute to worse health outcomes.

Financial Barriers and Lack of Insurance

Financial barriers are another major impediment to healthcare access in Black communities. Despite the Affordable Care Act's efforts to expand insurance coverage, Black Americans are still more likely to be uninsured than their white counterparts. According to the U.S. Department of Health and Human Services, 9.7% of Black Americans are uninsured compared to 5.4% of whites. The lack of health insurance makes it difficult for individuals to afford routine medical care, preventive services, and medications, leading to untreated conditions and a higher incidence of complications from chronic diseases.

Even for those with insurance, high out-of-pocket costs can deter individuals from seeking care. Co-pays, deductibles, and the cost of medications can be prohibitively expensive, particularly for low-income families. This financial strain forces many to forgo necessary medical visits, screenings, and treatments, exacerbating health issues that could have been managed or prevented with timely care.

Systemic Racism and Discrimination in Healthcare

Systemic racism within the healthcare system is a pervasive barrier that significantly impacts the quality of care received by Black individuals. Racism can manifest in many ways, from implicit bias in patient-provider interactions to structural inequalities in healthcare policies and practices. Studies have shown that Black patients are less likely to receive the same quality of care as white patients, even when controlling for factors such as income and insurance status. This inequity can lead to misdiagnoses, inadequate treatment, and a general mistrust of the healthcare system.

Discrimination in healthcare settings can also discourage Black individuals from seeking care. Experiences of racism, whether overt or subtle, can create a sense of alienation and fear, leading some to avoid medical visits altogether. This avoidance, coupled with the existing barriers to access, contributes to worsening health disparities.

Cultural Competency and Communication Barriers

Cultural competency among healthcare providers is crucial for delivering effective care to diverse populations. However, a lack of cultural understanding and sensitivity to healthcare can create significant barriers to care for Black patients. Miscommunication, cultural misunderstandings, and a lack of trust can result in patients not fully understanding their diagnoses, treatment options, or the importance of follow-up care. This can lead to poor adherence to treatment plans, lower satisfaction with care, and poorer health outcomes.

Healthcare providers who are not culturally competent may also fail to consider the social and cultural context of their patients' lives, leading to recommendations that are not feasible or appropriate for the patient's circumstances. For example, dietary advice that does not consider cultural food practices or economic constraints may be disregarded, leading to continued poor health outcomes.

Barriers to Preventive Care

Preventive care is essential for maintaining health and preventing the development of chronic diseases. However, Black communities face significant barriers to accessing preventive services. These barriers include a lack of insurance, financial constraints, and geographic limitations, as well as systemic issues such as racism and discrimination. Without access to preventive care, conditions that could be managed or even prevented through early intervention go undetected until they become more severe, requiring more complex and costly treatments.

Screening programs for conditions such as hypertension, diabetes, and cancer are less accessible to Black population, contributing to later-stage diagnoses and worse outcomes. For instance, Black women are more likely to be diagnosed with breast cancer at a later stage than white women, and Black men are more likely to be diagnosed with prostate cancer at a later stage than white men. These disparities in preventive care access highlight the need for targeted interventions to ensure all individuals have access to the screenings and services needed to maintain good health.

The Impact of Healthcare Infrastructure and Policy

Healthcare infrastructure and policy decisions play a significant role in perpetuating disparities. Hospitals and clinics in Black neighborhoods are often underfunded and understaffed, leading to longer times of waiting, fewer available services, and lower overall quality of care. Additionally, healthcare policies that do not adequately address the unique needs of Black communities can further entrench disparities. For example, Medicaid expansion under the Affordable Care Act has helped reduce the uninsured rate among low-income individuals. Still, many states with large Black population have opted not to expand Medicaid, leaving millions without coverage.

Public health initiatives and healthcare policies must be designed with an understanding of the specific barriers faced by Black communities. This includes ensuring that funding is allocated to improve healthcare infrastructure in underserved areas, expanding access to insurance coverage, and implementing training programs to increase cultural competency among healthcare providers.

Breaking the Cycle: Toward Equitable Healthcare Access

Addressing the role of healthcare access and systemic barriers in perpetuating health disparities requires a comprehensive approach that includes policy changes, community engagement, and education. We must advocate for policies that expand access to affordable healthcare, improve the quality of care in underserved areas, and train healthcare providers to recognize and address their biases.

Community-based initiatives that bring healthcare services directly to Black neighborhoods can help bridge the gap in access. Mobile clinics, telehealth services, and partnerships with local organizations can provide much-needed care to those who cannot reach healthcare facilities. Education is also vital—by increasing health literacy and empowering individuals to advocate for their health, we can help reduce the impact of systemic barriers and improve health outcomes for the Black community.

As we close this chapter, it is essential to recognize that healthcare access is not just about the availability of services but also about the quality and equity of those services. It ensures that all individuals, regardless of race or socio-economic status, have access to high-quality, culturally competent care. This is fundamental to achieving health equity and improving the overall health of Black communities.

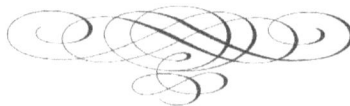

CHAPTER TWO

THE ROLE OF SOCIAL DETERMINANTS OF HEALTH

"Health isn't determined by genetics alone it's influenced by where we live, learn, work, and connect. To improve health, we must address these social factors at their roots."

SOCIAL DETERMINATIONS OF health refer to how people are born, grow, live, work, and age and how these factors influence overall health and well-being. Social determinants go beyond individual choices, highlighting how societal structures and systems impact access to care, health outcomes, and quality of life. For the Black community, these determinants play an outsized role in shaping health disparities.

Economic Stability

Economic stability is one of the most significant predictors of health. Individuals who live in stable economic environments have better access to essential health services, healthier living conditions, and the ability to make choices that promote long-term well-being. Unfortunately, many Black communities face economic instability stemming from systemic racism, historic underinvestment, and persistent unemployment.

Black Americans are disproportionately impacted by poverty, with almost 20% living below the poverty line, which limits access to nutritious food, healthcare, safe housing, and education. Economic instability forces families to prioritize immediate survival over long-term health, leading to food insecurity, delayed medical care, and limited opportunities for healthy living.

Economic security means more than just having a job—it includes access to resources such as affordable housing, safe neighborhoods, and financial services. Programs that address these issues, such as job training and financial literacy initiatives, can empower Black communities to build economic stability and improve their health outcomes.

Education

Education is a powerful determinant of health, with higher educational attainment leading to better health literacy, improved job prospects, and greater access to resources. Individuals with higher education levels tend to have more opportunities to make informed decisions about their health, have greater access to healthcare, and are better positioned to advocate for themselves in medical settings.

In Black communities, systemic inequities in education contribute to health disparities. Underfunded schools, lack of access to higher education, and fewer opportunities for economic mobility are barriers that prevent Black individuals from achieving optimal health outcomes. Health literacy is crucial in understanding and navigating the healthcare system, managing chronic diseases, and making informed decisions about health choices.

Investing in education, especially programs that target Black communities, is essential for addressing health disparities. Health education programs that equip individuals with the knowledge to prevent and manage diseases can significantly improve the overall health of these communities.

Social and Community Context

The social environment in which individuals live, including relationships, community support, and societal norms, also plays a crucial role in health outcomes. For the Black community, strong social networks and community engagement have historically provided essential support in times of hardship. However, systemic racism and structural inequalities can weaken these networks and contribute to stress, mental health issues, and diminished access to resources.

The importance of community health initiatives cannot be overstated. Programs that promote social cohesion, offer health education, and encourage community participation are vital in addressing health disparities. For instance, community centers that provide fitness classes, mental health support, and nutrition education empower individuals to take control of their health and create a culture of wellness within the community.

A keen sense of social belonging and support can mitigate some effects of economic hardship and lack of healthcare access. By fostering social connections and providing platforms for community engagement, Black communities can build resilience against the adverse health effects of systemic inequality.

Healthcare Access and Quality

Access to healthcare is fundamental to health outcomes, but it remains a significant barrier for many Black Americans. Healthcare access includes physical access to medical services and the quality of care received. Unfortunately, Black individuals often face multiple barriers to healthcare, including lack of insurance, high medical costs, and geographic inaccessibility.

In addition to physical access, the quality of care that Black Americans receive can be impacted by implicit bias and discrimination within the healthcare system. This leads to misdiagnoses, delayed treatment, and poorer outcomes compared to their white counterparts. Studies have shown that even when controlling for factors like income and education, Black patients often receive lower-quality care than white patients, highlighting the systemic inequities that persist in healthcare.

To address this, initiatives such as expanding Medicaid, increasing the number of Black healthcare professionals, and implementing culturally competent care are critical. Community health centers, telehealth services, and mobile clinics can also help bridge the gap by providing more accessible, affordable care to underserved Black population.

Unaddressed Determinants of Health

Health disparities in Black communities are influenced by a wide range of factors that extend beyond traditional social determinants. To comprehensively address these disparities, it is essential to consider additional elements such as environmental factors, food security, stress, and the impact of public policy. These factors, often intertwined with socio-economic and cultural determinants, play a critical role in shaping health outcomes and must be acknowledged and addressed in any efforts to promote health equity.

Environmental Factors

While we have previously touched on the impact of neighborhood safety and access to recreational spaces, it is essential to investigate deeper into the broader environmental challenges faced by Black communities. Many areas have prevalent ecological hazards such as pollution, inadequate housing, and lead exposure. These factors contribute to higher rates of respiratory diseases, developmental issues in children, and other chronic health conditions. Addressing these environmental injustices is crucial for creating healthier living conditions and reducing health disparities.

Food Security and Nutrition

Food security, defined as the availability of and access to nutritious food, is a critical yet often overlooked determinant of health. Many Black communities are in food deserts, where access to fresh, healthy food is limited. This lack of access leads to poor nutrition, which is linked to the prevalence of diet-related chronic diseases such as obesity, diabetes, and heart disease. By promoting community initiatives like urban farming, food cooperatives, and nutrition education, we can help improve food security and foster healthier eating habits.

The Impact of Stress and Mental Health

While we have discussed the cultural factors impacting mental health, it is also vital to recognize the role of chronic stress driven by socio-economic challenges and systemic racism. This chronic stress significantly impacts both physical and mental health, contributing to conditions such as hypertension, cardiovascular disease, depression, and anxiety. A holistic approach to health must address these stressors and promote access to culturally competent mental health services to support the Black population effectively.

The Role of Policy and Advocacy

Public policy has been a recurring theme in this book, particularly regarding healthcare access. However, it is equally important to consider how policies affecting social determinants such as income inequality, housing, and education can shape health outcomes. Advocacy efforts are essential for pushing for equitable policies that address these broader determinants of health. Individuals and communities can influence policy decisions that directly impact their health and well-being by engaging in advocacy.

Intersectionality and Vulnerable Populations

Finally, exploring the concept of intersectionality how overlapping identities such as race, gender, and socio-economic status influence health outcomes provides a deeper understanding of the unique challenges faced by individuals within the Black community. Addressing these intersecting identities is crucial for developing targeted interventions that effectively reduce health disparities across vulnerable populations.

Seven Lessons to Make *My Health, My Priority* a Reality

As we close this foundational section of the book, we must pause and reflect on the key insights we have uncovered together. These are not just observations lessons we can all take to heart as we strive to improve our health, communities, and lives. What follows are some reflections that I hope will resonate with you and inspire action.

1. Personal Experiences Shape Broader Understanding

Our personal stories hold incredible power. They help us understand the challenges we face and the resilience we muster to overcome them. My journey from a quiet childhood in Bamenda to balancing love, family, and ambition is not unique it is a story many of us can relate to in diverse ways. However, through these shared experiences, we can better understand the broader issues of health disparities and social challenges. Remember that our stories are not just our own; they are part of a larger narrative that can drive change and foster understanding.

2. Everything is Connected

We have seen how deeply interconnected the factors affecting our health are economic stability, education, social support, and healthcare access all play crucial roles. It is easy to feel overwhelmed by these complexities, but it is also empowering to recognize that by addressing one area, we can make positive changes in others. Our health is not just a matter of personal choice; the world influences it. By acknowledging these connections, we can take more informed steps toward improving our well-being.

3. Overcoming Barriers Requires Systemic Change

The challenges we face in accessing quality healthcare are not just about individual circumstances they are rooted in more significant systemic issues. Racism, discrimination, and structural inequalities create barriers that many of us struggle to overcome. It is important to recognize that personal effort is essential; progress requires systemic change. We must advocate for policies and practices that ensure everyone can access the care they need. Let us work together to break down these barriers so that all of us can thrive.

4. Cultural and Social Context Matters

Our cultural backgrounds and the communities we are part of shape our perceptions of health and influence our behaviors. What we have explored here is a reminder that culturally competent care is not a luxury but a necessity. Healthcare providers must understand and respect our diverse experiences to offer adequate care. But this also means that we, as individuals, must stay connected with our cultural roots and community support systems. These connections are powerful tools for maintaining our health and well-being.

5. Holistic Approaches Are Key

Addressing health disparities is not just about treating diseases it is about seeing the whole person. Our lives are complex, and many factors beyond the physical influence our health. We have discussed the importance of looking at the broader picture considering mental, emotional, and social health alongside physical health. Let us commit to embracing holistic approaches in our lives and communities, ensuring that we support each other in all aspects of health.

6. Advocacy and Empowerment Drive Change

Finally, we have learned that real change comes from empowerment and advocacy. Whether standing up for minorities or vulnerable ones in the doctor's office, educating members in the Black communities, or pushing for policy changes, we all have a role to play in creating a healthier future. Knowledge is power, but action turns that power into progress. Let us take what we have learned here and use it to advocate for better health for ourselves, our families, and our Black communities.

7. The Power of Community Engagement

One of the most important takeaways from our discussions is the power of community in shaping health outcomes. Individual efforts are crucial, but our impact is magnified when we come together as the Black community. Engaging with neighbors, sharing knowledge, and supporting one another in our health journeys are all vital components of building a healthier future.

Collective action whether through local health initiatives, community education programs, or simply checking in on one another can drive notable change. Let us remember that prioritizing health is not just a personal mission but a communal one. Lifting each other ensures that everyone in the Black community can thrive.

I hope you will carry these lessons as we progress in this book. They are not just my reflections our shared insights gained through understanding, empathy, and a commitment to making a difference. Together, we can build a future where health disparities are outdated, and everyone can live a healthy, fulfilling life. Let us practice healthy habits to prioritize our health with hope, determination, and purpose, knowing that our work today will create a healthier Black community.

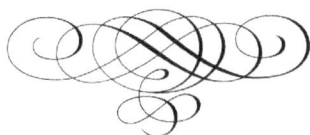

PART TWO

PREVENTION AND HEALTH MAINTENANCE

CHAPTER THREE

THE IMPORTANCE OF PREVENTIVE CARE

"Preventive care is the foundation of a healthy life by taking action today, we can prevent the illnesses of tomorrow and build stronger, more resilient communities."

AS WE EXPLORED IN PART ONE, the Black community faces significant health disparities that are deeply rooted in socio-economic, cultural, and systemic factors. Understanding these disparities is crucial, but our action to address them is equally important. This is where preventive care becomes essential. Preventive care is more than just a notion it is a proactive approach to managing health that can significantly reduce the risk of developing chronic conditions like diabetes, heart disease, and hypertension, which we identified as prevalent in the Black community.

Definitions and Benefits of Preventive Care

Preventive care involves routine check-ups, vaccinations, screenings, and lifestyle modifications that help stop health problems before they start. As we discussed earlier, chronic diseases often take hold when they go undetected or are not appropriately managed. By focusing on preventive care, we can shift from a reactive approach, which treats illnesses after they have developed, to a proactive approach that keeps us healthier and longer.

The benefits of preventive care are manifold and promising. Individuals can significantly reduce their risk of developing severe health conditions by using regular preventive practices. This foresight in maintaining good health can lead to long-term benefits, offering hope for a healthier future. For instance, regular screenings for conditions like hypertension and diabetes which are more prevalent in the Black community can lead to early detection, allowing for timely intervention and effective management. This eventually helps reduce healthcare costs by minimizing the need for expensive treatments and hospitalizations often resulting from advanced diseases.

Besides, preventive care is critical in enhancing the quality of life. By maintaining good health and catching potential issues early, individuals can avoid the physical and emotional toll of chronic diseases, which, as we have seen, disproportionately affect Black communities. Preventive care increases life expectancy and well-being, allowing everyone to lead healthier lives.

Preventive care is critical in the context of our discussions on health disparities. It represents a tangible way to close the gaps in health outcomes identified in Part One. By prioritizing preventive measures, members of the Black community can work towards ensuring that they can all live healthy, fulfilling lives. This aim resonates deeply with the mission of this book.

Preventive care also involves identifying risk factors and proactively mitigating them. As we saw earlier, understanding one's family health history can be a powerful tool in preventing the recurrence of common familial diseases. Suppose a person knows that diabetes runs in their family.

In that case, they can take preventive actions such as improving diet quality, managing weight, increasing physical activity, and undergoing regular medical check-ups, including diabetes screening and blood glucose monitoring. By taking these steps, individuals can significantly lower their risk of developing chronic conditions, demonstrating the tangible benefits of preventive care.

The emphasis on preventive care is about personal health and empowering our entire community. Just as we discussed the importance of education and awareness in earlier chapters, preventive care is another critical strategy in our collective effort to improve health outcomes for all.

How Preventive Care Can Reduce the Prevalence of Chronic Diseases

Chronic diseases such as hypertension, diabetes, and heart disease disproportionately affect the Black community. These conditions are often preventable through regular screenings, healthy lifestyle choices, and early intervention. Preventive care is essential in reducing the prevalence of these diseases by identifying risk factors early and implementing strategies to mitigate them.

For instance, regular blood pressure checks can help detect hypertension in its preliminary stages, allowing for timely intervention through lifestyle changes or medication. Similarly, blood glucose screenings can identify prediabetes, enabling individuals to take steps to prevent the progression to full-blown diabetes. By catching these conditions early, preventive care not only improves individual health outcomes but also reduces the overall burden of chronic diseases within the Black community.

Preventive care can also reduce the prevalence of diseases within a family and the broader Black community when individuals take proactive steps to eliminate risk factors. For example, a person with a family history of heart disease who engages in regular medical check-ups and adheres to a medical regimen is more likely to prevent the development of heart problems that are common in their family lineage.

If a person knows that heart disease runs in their family a grandfather had heart disease, followed by a father, and then a sibling they are at a higher risk of developing the condition themselves. However, being aware of this family history allows them to take prompt action, such as adopting a healthier lifestyle and seeking regular medical advice, to prevent the reoccurrence of such diseases.

In addition to screenings, preventive care includes education on healthy lifestyle choices. This can involve counseling on nutrition, physical activity, and avoiding harmful habits such as smoking and excessive alcohol consumption. When individuals are informed and empowered to make healthy choices, they are better equipped to prevent the onset of chronic diseases. By understanding and addressing the specific health risks within their families, individuals can make informed decisions that protect their health and contribute to the well-being of the entire Black community.

Role of Regular Check-ups and Screenings

Regular check-ups and screenings are the cornerstone of preventive care. These routine visits to healthcare providers allow for the early detection of potential health issues, even before symptoms appear. Regular check-ups enable healthcare providers to assess overall health, monitor vital signs, and recommend necessary screenings based on age, gender, family history, and lifestyle factors.

For the Black community, where access to healthcare and trust in the healthcare system may be barriers, regular check-ups are even more critical. These visits can build relationships with healthcare providers, increasing confidence and ensuring that individuals receive consistent, personalized care. Screenings such as mammograms, colonoscopies, and blood tests are vital tools in catching diseases like cancer, heart disease, and diabetes in their initial stages when they are most treatable.

Preventive measures, such as regular check-ups and screenings, are essential in reducing health problems within the Black community. The saying "prevention is better than cure" especially applies to chronic health conditions. There are several annual check-ups recommended for both men and women to help prevent diseases like cancer, heart disease, hypertension, and diabetes. Children, too, require regular screenings to prevent chronic diseases that may run in the family or other risk factors. Early detection of certain diseases enables timely intervention, allowing for the initiation of treatment before the disease progresses, thereby preventing the condition from worsening.

Regular check-ups offer an opportunity to discuss health concerns, receive vaccinations, and get advice on maintaining a healthy lifestyle. By prioritizing these routine visits, individuals can avoid potential health problems and take proactive steps toward long-term wellness.

Building a Preventive Care Routine and Overcoming Barriers

Establishing a preventive care routine involves incorporating regular healthcare visits, screenings, and healthy habits into everyday life. However, building and maintaining such a routine can be challenging due to various barriers, including financial constraints, lack of access to healthcare, and cultural factors.

Despite the well-documented benefits of preventive care, it is often overlooked, particularly in the Black community. Studies have shown that Black individuals are less likely to use preventive health services compared to their white counterparts. According to Donald M., Richard S., et al., one of the primary reasons for this disparity is the mistrust that many Black individuals have towards healthcare providers, which prevents them from seeking preventive care. This mistrust, rooted in historical and ongoing injustices, such as the infamous Tuskegee Syphilis Study, where Black men were deceived and denied treatment, continues to influence attitudes towards healthcare.

In the Black community, for example, many people are hesitant to take vaccines due to fears that they are part of a sinister agenda. There is a pervasive belief that healthcare providers may be using them as experimental subjects, a sentiment that stems from a long history of exploitation and abuse. This fear and mistrust hinder the adoption of preventive measures such as vaccinations, screenings, and regular check-ups, which are crucial for maintaining health and preventing diseases.

To overcome these barriers, it is essential to educate the Black community on the importance of preventive care and provide resources that make it accessible to all. Informal education, such as community workshops, can be an effective tool in spreading information about the benefits of preventive healthcare. Community health programs that offer free or low-cost screenings, educational workshops on healthy living, and partnerships with local healthcare providers can help increase access to preventive services and build trust within the community.

Financial barriers can also be addressed through health insurance programs that cover preventive care services at little to no cost. It is crucial to educate individuals about their insurance benefits and encourage them to take advantage of these services. For many, the cost of healthcare can be a significant obstacle, but by making preventive care more affordable, we can encourage more people to engage in these vital health practices.

Cultural barriers, such as mistrust of the healthcare system, can be mitigated by fostering relationships between healthcare providers and the Black community. Culturally competent care that respects and understands the unique needs and experiences of the Black community can help build trust and encourage individuals to engage in preventive care. Beyond just taking vaccines, yearly check-ups, regular exercise, a healthy diet, and avoiding harmful habits like smoking are all measures that can prevent diseases and promote overall well-being.

Conclusion: Embrace Preventive Care for a Healthier Future

As discussed in this chapter, preventive care is not just an individual responsibility but a collective effort that can transform the health of the Black communities. From regular check-ups and screenings to making informed lifestyle choices, preventive care provides us with the tools to stay ahead of chronic diseases and maintain our overall well-being.

We have seen that the Black community faces unique challenges when accessing and trusting healthcare services. However, by taking proactive steps—whether through education, building trust with healthcare providers, or advocating for better access to services—we can begin to close the gaps in health outcomes that have persisted for far too long.

Preventive care is about more than just avoiding illness; it is about fostering a culture of health and wellness that empowers us to live longer, fuller lives. By prioritizing our health and encouraging our loved ones to do the same, we set the foundation for a healthier future for ourselves and future generations.

While preventive care lays the groundwork for a healthy life, daily choices play an equally crucial role in shaping long-term health outcomes. The next chapter will examine the importance of healthy lifestyle choices focusing on diet, nutrition, physical activity, and avoiding harmful habits. Understanding and implementing these practices can enhance our well-being and reduce the risk of chronic diseases, reinforcing our commitment to prioritizing our health.

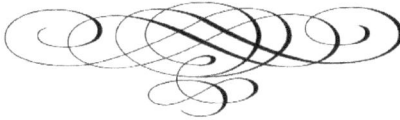

CHAPTER FOUR

HEALTHY LIFESTYLE CHOICES

"Healthy lifestyle choices are the building blocks of a vibrant life; each decision we make today shapes the strength of our tomorrow."

GIVEN THAT BLACK INDIVIDUALS are disproportionately affected by healthcare disparities such as limited access to care, implicit bias, and higher rates of chronic diseases like stroke, hypertension, and diabetes it is essential for the Black community to embrace preventive health measures. This includes proper nutrition, regular physical activity, avoiding unhealthy habits, and utilizing available health education resources.

Every time I read studies, such as those by William J.H., Kent M.L., et al. source and the Harvard School of Public Health source, which show that Black individuals suffer more health problems, are less likely to access healthcare and have higher death rates than other racial groups, it deeply concerns me. I am passionate about bringing health equity to the Black community and closing the gaps in disease prevalence between Black individuals and other races. The high rates of health disparities and shorter life expectancy among Black populations are issues that must be addressed. Choosing healthy lifestyle options is a significant first step forward.

Diet and Nutrition

Our journey towards better health begins with what we nourish our bodies daily. Diet and nutrition are fundamental components of a healthy lifestyle, serving as the foundation for overall well-being; what we eat impacts our physical, mental, and emotional states, influencing everything from energy levels to disease prevention.

Importance of a Balanced Diet

A balanced diet is essential for building a healthy body, preventing nutritional deficiencies, and consuming essential vitamins and minerals. It also serves as a means of disease prevention, helping to ward off conditions such as obesity, diabetes, and heart disease. A balanced diet involves consuming the right proportions of different food groups fruits, vegetables, whole grains, proteins, and healthy fats each uniquely supporting the body's functions.

One practical guide to a balanced diet is the "MyPlate" model, which emphasizes the importance of including various food groups vegetables, grains, dairy, protein, and fruits on your plate at each meal. The goal of "MyPlate" is to help individuals select the proper nutrition based on their body's requirements, promote better health, and prevent disorders such as obesity.

However, it is essential to acknowledge that achieving a balanced diet is not without challenges, particularly when considering socioeconomic factors like income and housing. Accessing nutritious food can be a significant struggle for many individuals, especially those facing homelessness or other financial hardships. As a healthcare provider, I work with patients who suffer from chronic conditions like diabetes, heart failure, and renal failure and who often struggle to have even a single meal a day. Despite these challenges, a balanced diet remains critical. Even in difficult circumstances, eating the right foods can help prevent further health deterioration, support disease prevention, and promote overall well-being.

Understanding and embracing the importance of a balanced diet is particularly critical. Historically, dietary habits have been shaped by cultural, economic, and social factors, which sometimes lead to imbalanced nutrition. Traditional diets, while rich in flavor and cultural significance, can often be high in fats, sugars, and sodium, contributing to higher rates of hypertension, diabetes, and obesity.

Transitioning to a balanced diet does not mean abandoning cultural foods but adapting them to be healthier. Incorporating more fruits, vegetables, and whole grains into traditional meals can significantly reduce the risk of chronic diseases. For instance, replacing refined grains with whole grains or adding more leafy greens to meals can boost nutrient intake without compromising taste.

Recognizing portion control and the importance of moderation is vital. Overeating, even healthy foods, can lead to weight gain and other health issues. By practicing mindful eating paying attention to what we eat, how much we eat, and how it makes us feel we can develop healthier eating habits that support long-term well-being.

Vitamin D Deficiency

Vitamin D is a crucial nutrient that supports bone health, immune function, and overall well-being. From my personal experience, I have seen how Vitamin D deficiency can significantly impact health. Vitamin D plays a vital role in helping the body absorb calcium into the bones, and without adequate Vitamin D, bone health can suffer due to poor calcium absorption.

Vitamin D deficiency is alarmingly common, especially among Black individuals. One of the primary reasons for this deficiency is the presence of melanin in the skin, which reduces the skin's ability to produce Vitamin D from sunlight. This makes it harder for people with darker skin to get enough Vitamin D naturally from sun exposure. Other contributing factors include poor nutrition, lack of access to healthcare, and knowledge deficits about the importance of Vitamin D.

From experience, I know many people are unaware of Vitamin D's critical role in overall health. This deficiency has been linked to a range of health problems, including osteoporosis, increased susceptibility to infections, and even certain chronic diseases such as cardiovascular disease and diabetes. Maintaining adequate Vitamin D levels is essential to prevent these issues.

Vitamin D supplementation can be a simple and effective solution for at-risk people. Additionally, incorporating Vitamin D-rich foods into the diet such as milk, fortified cereals, egg yolks, and certain types of fish like tuna can help boost levels naturally. Regularly outdoors in the sunlight, even for short periods, can also contribute to maintaining healthy Vitamin D levels, although it is crucial to balance sun exposure with skin protection.

Educating the community about the risks and prevention of Vitamin D deficiency is vital for promoting better health outcomes. By addressing this common yet often overlooked issue, we can take another step towards closing the health disparities gaps and ensuring everyone can lead a healthy, vibrant life.

Physical Activity

Physical activity is a cornerstone of a healthy lifestyle and is crucial in maintaining overall well-being. It is about exercise and any activity involving body movement, contributing to disease prevention and health maintenance. Engaging in regular physical activity helps prevent a sedentary lifestyle, which is associated with increased health risks such as blood clots, obesity, stroke, and contractures.

Benefits of Regular Exercise

Regular exercise offers numerous benefits that extend far beyond weight management. It is a powerful tool for preventing and managing chronic conditions such as hypertension, diabetes, and heart disease—ailments that disproportionately affect the Black community. Physical activity is essential in maintaining healthy body functions and preventing diseases like obesity, cardiovascular diseases, and type 2 diabetes. It also helps to relieve stress and improve overall mental health.

Physical activities can be achieved through various means, including walking, bicycling, sports, and dancing. For bedridden individuals, physical activity can be achieved through motion exercises. These activities contribute to physical health and significantly preserve mental health, relieve stress, and improve moods. When I start feeling exhausted and burned out, I know my body needs exercise.

In addition to the benefits above, regular exercise offers several other significant advantages:

Improved Immune System Function

Regular physical activity can boost the immune system, helping the body ward off illnesses and infections more effectively. This is particularly important for maintaining overall health and reducing the likelihood of frequently falling ill.

Enhanced Brain Health and Cognitive Function

Exercise has been shown to improve brain function, enhancing memory, concentration, and learning abilities. It also reduces the risk of cognitive decline and neurodegenerative diseases such as Alzheimer's disease.

Better Sleep Quality

Regular physical activity can help regulate sleep patterns, leading to better-quality sleep. Exercise promotes more profound and restful sleep, essential for overall health and well-being.

Increased Longevity

Regular exercise is associated with a longer life expectancy. By reducing the risk of chronic diseases and improving overall health, exercise contributes to a longer, healthier life.

Improved Digestive Health

Physical activity stimulates digestion and helps maintain a healthy gut. Regular exercise can reduce the risk of digestive issues such as constipation and irritable bowel syndrome (IBS).

Enhanced Flexibility and Mobility

Exercise, particularly stretching and flexibility routines, helps maintain and improve flexibility and joint mobility. This is essential for maintaining independence and preventing injuries as one ages.

Stronger Muscles and Bones

Weight-bearing exercises like resistance training help build and maintain muscle mass and bone density, reducing the risk of osteoporosis and fractures.

Social Interaction and Community Building

Participating in group sports or fitness classes provides opportunities for social interaction, fostering a sense of community and improving mental health through social support.

Enhanced Metabolic Rate

Regular physical activity increases the body's metabolic rate, which helps with weight management and maintaining a healthy body composition.

Reduced Risk of Certain Cancers

Exercise has been linked to a reduced risk of developing certain types of cancer, including breast, colon, and lung cancer.

According to the American Heart Association, 150 minutes of moderate-intensity aerobic activity or 75 minutes of vigorous-intensity aerobic activity per week is recommended to maintain good health. These guidelines emphasize the importance of regular physical activity in promoting overall well-being and preventing chronic diseases.

Types of Physical Activities Recommended

When it comes to physical activity, variety is vital. Incorporating diverse types of exercise into a routine can help target various fitness aspects, including strength, endurance, flexibility, and balance. Here are some recommended types of physical activities:

✱ Aerobic Exercises

Activities such as walking, running, cycling, swimming, and dancing fall into this category. Aerobic exercises are excellent for cardiovascular health, as they help to strengthen the heart and lungs, improve circulation, and boost overall energy levels.

✳ Strength Training

This involves exercises that build muscle strength and endurance, such as weightlifting, resistance band exercises, or bodyweight exercises like push-ups and squats. Strength training is essential for maintaining muscle mass, improving bone density, and enhancing metabolic function.

✳ Flexibility and Stretching Exercises

Activities like yoga, Pilates, and simple stretching routines help to improve flexibility, enhance range of motion, and prevent injuries. Flexibility exercises also promote relaxation and can help reduce stress.

✳ Balance Exercises

These exercises are fundamental as we age, helping to prevent falls and improve stability. Balance exercises include tai chi, balance drills, and exercises that focus on core strength.

Making Physical Activity a Part of Daily Life

Incorporating physical activity into daily life does not require a gym membership or fancy equipment. Simple changes, such as taking the stairs instead of the elevator, walking or cycling instead of driving short distances, and setting aside time each day for a brisk walk or a home workout, can make a significant difference.

If you face barriers to traditional forms of exercise, finding culturally relevant and enjoyable activities is critical.

Dancing to your favorite music, joining a local sports team, or participating in group fitness classes can make exercise feel less like a chore and more like a fun, social activity.

The most important aspect is consistency. It is not about doing intense daily workouts but making regular physical activity a habit. Over time, these small, consistent efforts add significant health benefits, helping reduce the risk of chronic diseases and improve overall quality of life.

Avoiding Harmful Habits

Living a healthy life is not just about adopting positive behaviors like eating well and exercising regularly; it is also about consciously avoiding habits that can cause harm to your body and mind. Certain behaviors, such as smoking, excessive alcohol consumption, and drug use, pose significant risks to your health and can undermine the benefits of even the healthiest routines.

As a healthcare worker, I have witnessed the dangers of smoking and alcohol abuse, which are significant contributors to the cause of death for many individuals. I have seen people suffer and die from health complications related to alcohol abuse. Harmful lifestyles, such as smoking and alcohol abuse, are major risk factors for chronic health problems like cardiovascular diseases, cancer, and stroke. The importance of avoiding unhealthy habits like smoking and alcohol abuse cannot be overstated.

Cigarette smoking is far more dangerous than many realize. According to the CDC, smoking causes approximately 480,000 deaths per year in the United States more than the deaths related to HIV, alcohol use, and illegal drugs combined. Additionally, nine out of ten lung cancer-related deaths and eight out of 10 Chronic Obstructive Pulmonary Disease (COPD)-related deaths are caused by cigarette smoking. (Source: CDC).

Studies also show that Black individuals have the highest rate of lung cancer related to smoking compared to any other race (Vani S. N., Barbara P., et al.)

The Dangers of Smoking and Vaping

Smoking remains one of the leading causes of preventable death worldwide. The harmful effects of smoking are well-documented, including an increased risk of lung cancer, heart disease, stroke, Chronic Obstructive Pulmonary Disease (COPD), and numerous other severe health conditions. In addition to these direct effects, secondhand smoke poses significant health risks to those around you, particularly children and individuals with pre-existing health conditions.

Vaping, often perceived as a safer alternative to smoking, is also associated with significant health risks. While vaping products do not contain tobacco, they still deliver nicotine and other harmful chemicals to the body, which can lead to addiction and other health issues. The long-term effects of vaping are still being studied, but there is growing evidence that it can cause lung damage and increase the risk of respiratory diseases.

For the Black community, smoking and vaping are concerning due to higher rates of tobacco use and the presence of other compounding factors, such as limited access to healthcare and lower rates of smoking cessation success. These habits contribute to the prevalence of chronic diseases like hypertension and heart disease, which can be avoided.

The Impact of Excessive Alcohol Consumption

Excessive alcohol consumption is another behavior that can have devastating effects on your health. While moderate alcohol consumption may not be harmful to some, excessive drinking can lead to a range of severe health issues, including liver disease, cardiovascular problems, mental health disorders, and an increased risk of accidents and injuries. Long-term excessive drinking can also lead to alcohol dependence, which can have far-reaching consequences for individuals and their families.

In the Black community, alcohol-related health issues are compounded by social and economic factors that can make it more difficult to access treatment and support for alcohol dependency. Cultural attitudes towards drinking may sometimes downplay the risks associated with alcohol use, making it harder to recognize when drinking has become a problem.

The Importance of Addressing Drug Use

Drug use, including the misuse of prescription medications, is a significant issue that can lead to addiction, overdose, and other serious health consequences. The misuse of drugs, whether illegal substances or prescription medications, poses a direct threat to both physical and mental health. The opioid crisis has had a devastating impact on communities across the United States, including the Black community.

Drug addiction often starts to cope with stress, trauma, or other life challenges. Still, it quickly spirals into a destructive cycle that affects not only the individual but also their family and community. Access to treatment and support is crucial for those struggling with addiction, and it is essential to recognize the signs of drug misuse early to prevent further harm.

Tips for Quitting and Reducing Intake

Quitting smoking, reducing alcohol intake, and avoiding drug use are some of the most impactful steps you can take to improve your health. While these changes can be challenging, they are achievable with the right strategies and support. To successfully quit smoking, individuals may need social support, nicotine patches, or therapy, and it is essential to be intentional about the decision to leave.

Reducing alcohol intake and consuming it in moderation is also crucial. To avoid withdrawal symptoms, it is advisable to decrease alcohol consumption gradually. Seeking support from groups like Alcoholics Anonymous (AA) can provide valuable assistance to others who have faced similar challenges in overcoming unhealthy habits. It is also important to avoid places, groups, or friends who are not supportive of your decision to quit.

For quitting smoking and vaping:

* Set a Quit Date

Choose a quit date within the next two weeks. This will give you enough time to prepare but keep the goal within reach.

* Seek Support

Tell friends, family, and coworkers that you plan to quit and ask for their support. Consider joining a smoking cessation program or seeking counseling.

* Consider Nicotine Replacement Therapy (NRT)

NRT options like patches, gum, or lozenges can help reduce withdrawal symptoms and cravings, making it easier to quit.

* Avoid Triggers

Identify the situations that make you want to smoke or vape, and plan how to deal with them without turning to nicotine.

✳ Stay Busy

Engage in activities that keep your hands and mind occupied, helping you resist the urge to smoke or vape.

For reducing alcohol intake:

✳ Set Limits

Decide how many drinks you will have in a day or week and stick to it. Keeping track of your drinking can help you stay within your limits.

✳ Drink Slowly

Sip your drinks slowly and alternate alcoholic beverages with water or other non-alcoholic options.

✳ Avoid Binge Drinking

If you choose to drink, avoid consuming enormous quantities in a brief period, which can lead to serious health risks.

✳ Choose Alcohol-Free Days

Designate certain days of the week as alcohol-free to give your body a break and reduce your overall intake.

✳ Seek Help if Needed.

If you find it difficult to control your drinking, consider talking to a healthcare provider or joining a support group.

For addressing drug use:

✻ Recognize the Signs

Be aware of the signs of drug misuse, including changes in behavior, mood swings, and neglect of responsibilities.

✻ Seek Professional Help

If you or someone you know is struggling with drug addiction, seek professional help as soon as possible. Early intervention can prevent the problem from worsening.

✻ Build a Support Network

Surround yourself with people who support your decision to avoid drugs and encourage healthy habits.

✻ Stay Informed

Educate yourself and others about the risks of drug use and the importance of seeking help when needed.

Building and Maintaining Healthy Habits for Long-Term Wellness

Adopting healthy habits is essential for achieving long-term wellness. Still, it is not just about making changes for a brief period—it's about creating a sustainable lifestyle that promotes ongoing health and well-being. Building and maintaining these habits requires commitment, consistency, and a supportive environment encouraging positive behaviors.

Getting good rest and sleep is essential for building long-term wellness. Quality sleep allows the body to rest and recharge, which is crucial for overall health. I often tell my friends and colleagues that I prioritize getting enough rest because it helps me function better. Good rest rejuvenates the spirit and provides the strength needed for daily activities.

Regular exercise is another key component of maintaining a healthy lifestyle and long-term wellness. When I start feeling exhausted, burned out, or stressed, I know it is time for exercise. Physical activity revitalizes my entire being, whether I go for a walk or moderate exercise at a park. Exercise helps refresh the mind, body, and soul.

Eating right is also vital for disease prevention and maintaining good health. While a balanced diet is essential, eating at the right time is also important. I have noticed that many Africans do not pay much attention to meal timing. For example, eating late at night, sometimes around 9 or 10 p.m., and often in generous portions, is expected during social gatherings. Work schedules can also impact eating habits, especially for night shift workers who tend to eat during late hours.

To maintain and preserve a healthy well-being, it is essential to consider what you eat and when you eat. For

MIRANDA NDIFON NZOYEM

instance, choosing water over alcohol or sugary drinks is necessary for disease prevention and health maintenance. Water helps fight infection, regulates body temperature, and improves digestion. Even in hospitals, water is often the first line of treatment to fight infection. Eating more vegetables, fruits, and grains is also essential while reducing the intake of fatty foods.

Socialization is another aspect of building and maintaining a healthy lifestyle. While taking time alone to rest and recharge is important, it is equally essential to socialize occasionally. Giving and receiving love, laughter, and hugs can reduce stress and refresh the mind, body, and soul. Socialization and robust social support systems are vital for promoting overall well-being.

It is also crucial to use preventive care, such as yearly checkups and following doctors' recommendations. Vaccinations, such as those for hepatitis, pneumococcal disease, flu, and varicella, can boost immunity and improve health outcomes.

The Importance of Consistency in Healthy Habits

Consistency is the key to turning healthy choices into lasting habits. Whether it is regular physical activity, a balanced diet, or avoiding harmful habits, the benefits of these actions accumulate over time. Small, consistent efforts can lead to significant health improvements, whereas sporadic or inconsistent practices may yield different results.

To build consistency, setting realistic goals and creating a routine that fits into your daily life is essential. This might include scheduling regular exercise sessions, planning balanced meals ahead of time, or setting reminders to take breaks and relax. By incorporating these activities into your routine, they become second nature, eventually making it easier to maintain them.

Overcoming Barriers to Healthy Habits

Despite the best intentions, various barriers can make establishing and maintaining healthy habits challenging. These barriers can be physical, such as a lack of access to nutritious foods or safe spaces for exercise, or psychological, such as stress, lack of motivation, or emotional challenges.

It is crucial to identify these barriers early and develop strategies to overcome them. For example, if access to fresh produce is limited, consider growing your vegetables or finding affordable local markets. If time constraints make exercising hard, try incorporating physical activity into your daily routine—taking the stairs instead of the elevator, walking or biking to work, or doing short workouts at home.

Support systems play a vital role in overcoming barriers. Surround yourself with friends, family, or community members who encourage and support your healthy choices. Joining a group or community focused on health and wellness can provide motivation, accountability, and shared resources.

Creating a Supportive Environment

A supportive environment is essential for maintaining healthy habits. This includes the physical environment and your life's social and emotional aspects. This might mean keeping healthy snacks readily available, preparing meals in advance, and creating a space for exercise or relaxation at home.

Social support is equally important. Engaging with others who share similar health goals can foster a sense of community and encouragement. Whether participating in a fitness class, joining a support group, or simply sharing your journey with friends and family, having a support network can make it easier to stick to your healthy habits.

The Role of Mindset in Sustaining Healthy Habits

Your mindset plays a crucial role in the success of your health journey. Adopting a growth mindset—believing you can develop and improve your health through effort and persistence can make a significant difference. Instead of viewing challenges as setbacks, see them as opportunities to learn and grow.

It is also important to celebrate small victories along the way. Acknowledging progress, no matter how minor, reinforces your commitment and builds confidence in your ability to maintain healthy habits. Remember, wellness is a journey, not a destination; every step forward is a step toward better health.

Conclusion: Embrace Healthy Lifestyle Choices for Lasting Wellness

The foundation of a healthy life is the daily choices we make. Each element promotes long-term wellness, from balanced nutrition and regular physical activity to avoiding harmful habits and ensuring adequate rest.

Healthy lifestyle choices improve physical health and enhance mental, emotional, and social well-being. By prioritizing these habits, we can prevent chronic diseases, boost our energy levels, and enjoy a higher quality of life.

However, the journey toward wellness requires consistency, commitment, and a supportive environment. It is important to remember that small, consistent actions can lead to significant health benefits over time. Whether being available for exercise, choosing water over sugary drinks, or ensuring you get enough sleep, every positive step contributes to your overall well-being.

As we move forward, let us embrace these healthy lifestyle choices with intention and purpose. By doing so, we improve our health and set a powerful example for others, inspiring our community to prioritize health and wellness in their lives. Together, we can build a future where our health is our priority.

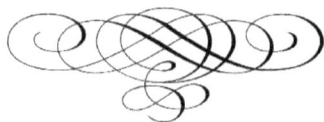

CHAPTER FIVE

MANAGING STRESS AND MENTAL HEALTH

"Taking care of our mental health is not just about surviving the pressures of today; it's about thriving in the possibilities of tomorrow."

STRESS IS A COMPLEX response that can manifest as feelings of exhaustion, excessive discomfort, or overwhelming pressure, whether from external or internal sources. When the body struggles to manage these challenges, stress can negatively impact our emotional, physical, and mental well-being. It weakens the immune system, making individuals more susceptible to infections, and can have far-reaching effects on overall health.

Uncontrolled stress can disrupt relationships, work life, and eating habits, leading to various health issues such as high blood pressure, poor blood sugar control, heart problems, and weight gain. In some cases, stress can drive individuals to engage in harmful behaviors like heavy drinking, smoking, or overeating, further exacerbating its detrimental impact on health and well-being.

It can result in physical symptoms like muscle tightness and stiffness, causing pain and discomfort. Personally, when I begin to experience tense back pain, I recognize it as a sign of stress, even if the specific stressor is not immediately apparent. This highlights the importance of proper stress management for disease prevention and health maintenance.

Impact of Stress on Physical Health

Stress is an inevitable part of life, but chronic stress can have severe consequences for physical health. Stress triggers a cascade of physiological responses in the body, including releasing stress hormones like cortisol. While these hormones are essential for responding to immediate threats, prolonged exposure can lead to a host of health problems.

Chronic stress has been linked to various physical ailments, including hypertension, heart disease, diabetes, and weakened immune function. For the Black community, where the added pressures of racial discrimination, economic challenges, and health disparities are prevalent, the impact of stress on physical health can be even more profound.

In my experience, I have noticed the unique challenges we face in our community, where socioeconomic factors and systemic inequalities often compound stress. These stressors do not just affect our physical health; they also contribute to the development of chronic conditions that disproportionately impact Africans or Black people.

Knowing the connection between stress and physical health is crucial for managing its effects. By recognizing the signs of chronic stress and taking proactive steps to address it, individuals can mitigate its impact on their health and well-being.

Techniques for Stress Management

Managing stress effectively requires a holistic approach that addresses the mind and body. Over time, I have learned the importance of using accessible and practical techniques to cope with stress. Deep breathing, relaxation exercises, meditation, listening to music, exercising, eating healthy foods, and engaging in social activities significantly reduce anxiety. These methods help relax the body by lowering blood pressure, reducing heart rate, stabilizing blood glucose levels, easing muscle tension, and decreasing pain.

Let us discover some of the most effective techniques for managing stress and how they can be integrated into your daily routine:

Mindfulness and Relaxation Exercises

Mindfulness involves staying present and observing thoughts and feelings without judgment. It helps reduce stress by increasing awareness of stressors and reactions to them. Techniques such as deep breathing, meditation, and progressive muscle relaxation are simple yet powerful tools that can be practiced anywhere.

Physical Activity

As discussed in previous chapters, regular exercise benefits physical health and stress management. Physical activity releases endorphins, which elevate mood and reduce stress. Incorporating movement into daily routines, whether through brisk walking, yoga, or dancing, is an effective way to manage stress.

Healthy Social Interactions

Connecting with others provides emotional support and can be a powerful stress reliever. Engaging in meaningful conversations, spending time with loved ones, or participating in group activities helps alleviate stress and fosters a sense of belonging.

Creative Outlets

Engaging in creative activities like art, music, writing, or gardening can serve as an outlet for stress and provide a sense of accomplishment. These activities offer a way to express oneself and distract from daily pressures.

Incorporating these techniques into your daily life can profoundly affect managing stress and maintaining overall well-being.

Importance of Mental Health and Seeking Help When Needed.

Mental health is just as crucial as physical health, yet it often does not receive the attention it deserves. Maintaining our mental well-being is essential for leading a balanced and fulfilling life. A healthy mental state helps us cope with external stress, build meaningful relationships, and make better and more nutritious choices.

Unfortunately, mental health is not a common topic discussed in many African communities. There is a cultural stigma attached to mental health disorders, making it difficult for many Black individuals to seek help. Mental health issues like depression, PTSD (Post Traumatic Stress Disorder), anxiety, and psychosis are real and have a significant impact on well-being. However, due to cultural beliefs, many Africans view mental health discussions as taboo and suggesting someone see a therapist can be seen as an insult.

This stigma prevents people from getting the help they need promptly. It is crucial to understand that mental health challenges are not a sign of weakness, and seeking help is a vital step in maintaining overall well-being. Mental health professionals, including therapists and counselors, can provide support and guidance through challenging times.

In my experience, maintaining mental health is essential for disease prevention and overall health maintenance. More exposure and awareness are needed in African communities so that everyone can benefit from professional help when needed. Remember, taking care of your mind is just as important as taking care of your body, and there is no shame in asking for help when you need it.

Building a Supportive Environment for Mental Well-Being

Creating a supportive environment is essential for maintaining mental well-being. The environment we live in, both physically and socially, plays a significant role in our mental health. A supportive environment provides a foundation for resilience, helping us to manage stress and navigate life's challenges more effectively.

Home Environment:

A peaceful and organized home can serve as a sanctuary from the stresses of the outside world. Creating a space where you feel safe and comfortable is crucial. This might involve decluttering, setting up areas dedicated to relaxation, and establishing boundaries between work and personal life. Ensuring your home is a place of rest and rejuvenation can significantly improve your mental health.

Social Support:

Surrounding yourself with positive, supportive people is vital for mental well-being. Strong relationships with family, friends, and community members provide emotional support, reduce feelings of loneliness, and offer valuable perspectives during tough times.

Engaging in social activities and building meaningful relationships based on trust and respect are essential for fostering a positive mental state. Furthermore, creating a life filled with purpose, passion, and aspiration further enhances mental well-being. It is necessary to seek mental health assistance to navigate challenges healthily when needed.

Community Engagement:

Being part of a community, whether through church, cultural organizations, or neighborhood activities, fosters a sense of belonging and provides a support system outside your immediate circle. Community engagement helps you feel connected and offers opportunities to contribute and find purpose, critical aspects of mental health.

Workplace Environment:

Managing stress in the workplace is crucial for overall mental health. This includes setting clear boundaries between work and personal life, taking regular breaks, and seeking support from colleagues or supervisors when needed. Promoting mental health awareness in the workplace can also contribute to a more supportive and understanding environment.

Access to Resources:

Ensuring access to mental health resources is critical for maintaining well-being. This includes knowing where to find help, accessing mental health services, and utilizing tools like therapy, counseling, and support groups. Educating yourself and others about available mental health resources can empower you to seek help when needed.

Building a supportive environment at home and in the community creates a solid foundation for mental well-being. It is vital to cultivate these supportive spaces actively, as they play a crucial role in managing stress and maintaining a healthy mind.

7 Lessons to Guide You in Prevention and Health Maintenance

While pondering Section Two, "Prevention and Health Maintenance," we have uncovered the power we hold over our well-being. Our expedition through this section has shown us that maintaining health is not just about reacting to issues as they arise but about proactively creating a life that prevents them. We have also explored the unique challenges the African community faces and the importance of supporting one another in overcoming barriers to healthcare and fostering environments that promote health.

The knowledge and insights we gained here laid a sturdy foundation for a healthier, more empowered future. Now, let us take a moment to distill these critical insights into actionable lessons that we can carry forward.

1. Prevention is the First Line of Defense

We have learned that taking preventive measures is crucial for avoiding the onset of chronic diseases. Regular check-ups, screenings, and healthy habits form the foundation of a life focused on wellness. By taking the initiative, we can catch potential health issues early and take steps to prevent them from developing into more severe conditions. Prevention is not just about avoiding illness it is about embracing a lifestyle that supports long-term health.

2. Healthy Choices Are Powerful

Our daily choices what we eat, move, and habits profoundly impact our overall health. We have discussed the importance of a balanced diet, regular physical activity, and avoiding harmful habits like smoking and excessive drinking. These choices are within our control and offer a powerful way to influence our well-being positively. Remember, every small decision contributes to a healthier future.

3. Stress Management is Essential

Stress is an unavoidable part of life, but how we manage it can make all the difference. Through mindfulness, physical activity, and social support, we can mitigate the adverse effects of stress on our physical and mental health. Effective stress management is not just about feeling better now—it is about protecting our health overall. Let us make stress management a priority, ensuring that we take care of our minds as well as our bodies.

4. Mental Health Deserves Our Attention

Mental health is often overlooked but is a critical component of overall well-being. We have discussed the importance of recognizing mental health challenges and seeking help when needed. Whether through professional support or leaning on our community, taking care of our mental health is essential for living a balanced life. Let us break the stigma and ensure that mental health is given the attention it deserves.

5. Build a Supportive Environment

Our physical and social environment plays a significant role in our health. Surrounding ourselves with positive influences, creating a peaceful home, and engaging in meaningful social interactions all contribute to our mental and physical well-being. A supportive environment helps us thrive, making maintaining healthy habits and managing stress easier. Let us be intentional about the environments we create for ourselves and our loved ones.

6. Empowerment Through Education

Knowledge is a powerful tool for health empowerment. We take control of our well-being by educating ourselves about preventive care, healthy lifestyle choices, and mental health. The information we have explored in this section serves as a foundation for making informed decisions that benefit our health. Let us continue to seek knowledge and use it to guide our healthy journeys.

7. Community Health is Our Collective Responsibility

Our health is interconnected with the health of our community. By prioritizing our well-being and encouraging others to do the same, we contribute to a healthier, stronger community. Whether through sharing knowledge, supporting local health initiatives, or simply being there for one another, our collective efforts can drive meaningful change. Let us remember that health is not just a personal mission it is a communal one, and together, we can have influence.

These are not just my thoughts they are the collective wisdom I have gathered through shared experiences, understanding, and a mutual commitment to bettering our health and communities through my career and networks. So far, you agree that we have the power to create a future where everyone has the chance to live a vibrant, healthy life. Let us embrace healthy choices against all odds, prioritizing our health with steadfast determination and a clear sense of purpose. Our choices today will pave the way for a brighter, healthier tomorrow for all of us.

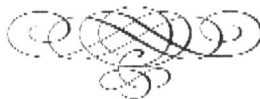

PART THREE

DISEASE-SPECIFIC PREVENTION AND MANAGEMENT

CHAPTER SIX

CARDIOVASCULAR DISEASES

"Our hearts beat not just for ourselves but for the strength and health of our entire community. To protect our hearts is to safeguard our collective future."

THE IMPORTANCE OF preventive care and healthy lifestyle choices emphasize that taking proactive steps is vital for maintaining our overall well-being. However, to truly make our health a priority, we must also understand the specific diseases that disproportionately affect the Black community and how we can manage them effectively.

This part of the book dips into the prevention and management of disease-specific conditions, focusing on those that pose the most significant risk to the health of Africans. By equipping ourselves with this knowledge, we can continue to take charge of our health for our benefit and the strength and vitality of the Black community. Let us start with:

Hypertension: The Silent Killer in the Black Community

Hypertension, often referred to as high blood pressure, is one of the most prevalent cardiovascular diseases among Black people. It is a condition where the force of blood against the artery walls is consistently too high, leading to severe health complications if left unmanaged. Despite its often-silent nature, hypertension is still a leading cause of untimely death worldwide, particularly affecting blacks at alarming rates.

The World Health Organization (WHO) defines hypertension as a blood pressure reading of 140/90 mmHg or higher, with an average level of around 120/80 mmHg. It is estimated that most adults in the African Community between the ages of 30-79 are living with hypertension, making it a significant health concern for Black people.

Studies have shown that the Black Community faces a higher prevalence of hypertension compared to other groups. Research highlights that Black people are more likely to develop high blood pressure, and managing this condition often requires a more aggressive and multifaceted approach. Biological differences play a crucial role in why hypertension is more common and more challenging to control among Africans.

As a healthcare provider, I have observed that Africans require more than one medication to manage blood pressure effectively. Calcium channel blockers and thiazide diuretics have been identified as particularly influential. However, it is essential to emphasize that treatment should be tailored to the individual rather than solely based on race to ensure the best possible outcomes.

One critical point I want to stress is the importance of taking blood pressure medications as prescribed. Many people may miss doses or stop taking their medications once they start feeling better, which can lead to severe complications such as stroke, heart failure, or kidney failure. Remember, most diseases like high blood pressure need lifelong management. Consistent medication use, along with regular monitoring, is vital to managing hypertension effectively.

Symptoms and Recommendations

Hypertension is often called a "silent killer" because it can develop without noticeable symptoms until significant damage has occurred. However, some common symptoms include severe headaches, chest pain, dizziness, breathing difficulties, abnormal heart rates, vision problems, and nosebleeds. Recognizing these symptoms and seeking prompt medical attention can prevent further complications.

For those diagnosed with or at risk of developing hypertension, I recommend keeping a healthy weight, adopting a heart-healthy diet rich in fruits, vegetables, and whole grains, reducing salt and processed food intake, limiting alcohol consumption, quitting smoking, and engaging in regular physical activity. These lifestyle changes can significantly help prevent or control hypertension.

Understanding Risk Factors

Hypertension can result from various factors, some of which we can control and others beyond our influence. Modifiable risk factors include poor diet, overweight, alcohol abuse, tobacco use, stress, and physical inactivity. We can change These behaviors and lifestyle choices to reduce our risk of developing high blood pressure.

Non-modifiable risk factors include genetics, family history, age, and race. It is essential to recognize that Africans tend to develop hypertension earlier than others, making awareness and early action crucial. Understanding our family health history can empower us to take proactive measures to reduce the likelihood of developing hypertension.

Given the disproportionate impact of hypertension in the Black community, Africans need to take responsibility for managing the risk factors within their control. Continuously seeking knowledge, asking questions, and having open discussions with primary healthcare providers are vital steps in staying informed and proactive about one's health.

Prevention is indeed better than cure, especially when managing hypertension, which can be particularly challenging. By prioritizing preventive care, adhering to treatment, and embracing healthier lifestyles, Africans can work together to reduce the burden of hypertension in the Black community and enhance better health for all.

Heart Failure: Understanding and Managing a Common Threat

Heart failure, another critical cardiovascular condition, is a chronic and progressive disease that significantly affects the African community. It occurs when the heart cannot pump blood efficiently enough to meet the body's needs, leading to shortness of breath, fatigue, and swelling in the legs and ankles.

Over time, this condition can severely impact a person's quality of life and, if left untreated, can be life-threatening. It is challenging to discuss cardiovascular diseases without addressing heart failure, especially given its alarming prevalence among Black people. According to studies, Black individuals have a 50% higher rate of heart failure compared to other races. This chronic condition occurs when the heart cannot pump blood effectively, leading to fluid buildup in different parts of the body, and it has far-reaching complications for our health.

This condition not only leads to a higher rate of hospitalizations but also results in worse clinical outcomes and is a leading cause of death among Africans. Given these severe risks, it is crucial for those of us at risk or already diagnosed with heart failure to be vigilant about our health.

Understanding the risk factors is a critical step in proactively preventing heart failure. These risk factors include hypertension, diabetes mellitus, obesity, high cholesterol, kidney failure, family history, an unhealthy diet, and smoking. For example, poorly controlled hypertension increases the workload of the heart, damaging the blood vessels and heart muscle. When the heart does not function properly, it can no longer pump blood effectively, leading to fluid buildup in various body parts.

The symptoms of heart failure vary depending on which side of the heart is affected. If the left side of the heart is compromised, individuals may experience respiratory issues such as fluid buildup in the lungs, difficulty breathing, coughing, or shortness of breath. If the right side of the heart is affected, symptoms may include swollen legs, a distended stomach (ascites), weight gain, a puffy appearance, and fatigue. Recognizing these symptoms early and seeking medical attention is essential to managing heart failure effectively.

It is also essential to consider the role of family history in heart failure. This condition often occurs in families, so understanding your family's health history is crucial. Even if the cause of heart failure is non-modifiable, being aware of this risk can empower you to adopt a healthier lifestyle, potentially delaying or preventing the onset of the disease.

In my clinical practice, I have observed with concern that heart failure tends to affect younger members of the African community more frequently than others. This raises questions about whether this is due to a lack of knowledge, unawareness, or other non-modifiable factors beyond control. Regardless of the cause, understanding these risks and taking proactive measures are essential for better health outcomes.

Recognizing the Symptoms of Heart Failure

Heart failure symptoms can vary from person to person, but some common signs include:

✳ Shortness of Breath

This can occur during physical activity, resting, or even lying down.

✳ Fatigue and Weakness

A feeling of constant tiredness or difficulty performing daily activities.

✳ Swelling (Edema)

Fluid buildup in the legs, ankles, or abdomen.

✳ Rapid or Irregular Heartbeat

A fast or fluttering heartbeat, which may be accompanied by chest pain.

✳ Persistent Coughing or Wheezing

Especially when lying down, which can be due to fluid buildup in the lungs.

Recognizing these symptoms early and seeking medical attention is essential for managing heart failure effectively. Early intervention can help slow the progression of the disease, improve quality of life, and reduce the risk of complications.

A Comprehensive Approach to Managing Heart Failure

Managing heart failure requires a multifaceted approach that includes lifestyle changes, medication, and regular monitoring. For many of us, this journey starts with making healthier lifestyle choices, such as:

Diet

Adopting a heart-healthy diet low in sodium, saturated fats, and sugars can help reduce the strain on the heart.

Exercise

Regular, moderate physical activity can strengthen the heart and improve cardiovascular health. Always consult with a healthcare provider to decide the proper level of activity.

Medications

Medications are often prescribed to help manage heart failure symptoms and prevent further damage to the heart. These may include diuretics, beta-blockers, ACE inhibitors, and others. Taking these medications as prescribed and having regular check-ups with a healthcare provider is crucial.

In addition to these measures, regular monitoring of symptoms and frequent visits to a healthcare provider is necessary to adjust treatment plans as needed. This ongoing care is vital to managing heart failure and preventing hospitalizations.

The Importance of Support Systems

Living with heart failure can be challenging, but it is essential to remember that we do not have to face it alone. Building a support system of family, friends, and healthcare providers can make a significant difference. Support groups, either in person or online, can also provide valuable resources and a sense of community for those managing heart failure.

Heart failure is a severe condition, but with proper care and support, it is possible to manage it effectively and keep a good quality of life. By staying informed, making healthy lifestyle choices, and working closely with healthcare providers, we can take control of our health and continue to live fulfilling lives despite the challenges posed by heart failure.

Monitoring and Managing Blood Pressure at Home

Monitoring and managing blood pressure at home is crucial for anyone diagnosed with hypertension or at high risk of developing it. Regularly tracking your blood pressure can help you manage your condition more effectively and prevent potential complications. It is not just about taking medications as prescribed; it is about understanding your body and being proactive in your health care.

For those of us on blood pressure medications, I strongly recommend checking your blood pressure before taking your medication each day. It is essential to consult your healthcare provider about the specific blood pressure range that would require you to hold off on taking your medication. This is because taking blood pressure medication when your blood pressure is already low can lead to dangerous drops, increasing the risk of falls and trauma; monitoring your blood pressure regularly while on medication helps you stay informed and make safe decisions about your treatment.

Normal blood pressure is around 120/80 mmHg. If your blood pressure is not well-controlled or if you are experiencing side effects from your medication, it is vital to speak with your healthcare provider. They can help adjust your medication or explore alternative treatments to ensure your blood pressure stays within a healthy range.

Besides watching your blood pressure, protecting your heart health requires adopting a heart-healthy lifestyle. This includes eating a balanced diet rich in fruits, vegetables, and whole grains while avoiding salty and oily foods. Maintaining a healthy weight, engaging in regular physical activity, and quitting smoking are critical steps in reducing the strain on your heart and improving your cardiovascular health. Limiting alcohol intake to a glass per day and keeping your blood glucose levels under control are equally important in managing blood pressure and preventing complications.

The Importance of Home Monitoring

Monitoring blood pressure at home lets you track your condition in real-time and make informed decisions about your health. It clarifies how your blood pressure fluctuates throughout the day and how it responds to different activities, foods, and medications. This real-time data is invaluable, especially since blood pressure readings taken in a clinical setting can sometimes be higher due to the stress or anxiety of being in a doctor's office—a phenomenon known as "white coat syndrome."

By regularly watching your blood pressure at home, you can:

* ★ Detect changes early.

Regular monitoring helps catch any unusual spikes or drops in blood pressure, allowing prompt intervention before they become a more serious issue.

* Assess the effectiveness of treatment.

Monitoring how your blood pressure responds to medications helps you and your healthcare provider decide whether your treatment plan works or needs adjustment.

* Encourage adherence to healthy habits.

The positive effects of lifestyle changes, such as diet and exercise, reflected in your blood pressure readings can motivate you to stick to these healthy habits.

Best Practices for Home Monitoring

To get the most exact and valuable information from home blood pressure monitoring, it is essential to follow these best practices:

* Use a reliable blood pressure monitor.

Invest in a good-quality, automated home blood pressure monitor. Wrist and finger monitors can be less exact, so an upper-arm monitor is recommended.

* Measure at the same time each day

Blood pressure fluctuates throughout the day, so it is important to take readings simultaneously each day, such as in the morning, before eating or taking medications.

★ Avoid caffeine, exercise, and smoking before measuring.

These can temporarily raise your blood pressure, leading to inaccurate readings. Aim to rest quietly for at least five minutes before taking a measurement.

★ Sit correctly.

Sit in a chair with your back supported and both feet flat on the floor. Rest your arm on a flat surface so your upper arm is at heart level. Avoid talking or moving during the measurement.

★ Take multiple readings.

Each time you measure, take two or three readings, one minute apart. Record the results and share them with your healthcare provider during check-ups.

Managing Hypertension Through Lifestyle Changes

Monitoring your blood pressure is only part of the equation. Lifestyle changes are essential to effectively managing hypertension.

These include:

Adopting a heart-healthy diet

A diet low in sodium, saturated fats, and cholesterol but rich in fruits, vegetables, whole grains, and lean proteins can significantly reduce blood pressure.

Regular physical activity

Aim for at least 150 minutes of moderate-intensity exercise, such as brisk walking, each week. Exercise strengthens the heart, allowing it to pump more efficiently with less effort.

Maintaining a healthy weight

Losing even a small amount of weight can significantly impact your blood pressure. Work with your healthcare provider to determine a healthy weight range.

Reducing alcohol intake

Drinking too much alcohol can raise blood pressure. If you drink alcohol, do so in moderation no more than one drink per day for women and two for men.

Quitting smoking

Smoking damages blood vessels and raises blood pressure. Quitting smoking is one of the best things you can do for your heart health.

Managing stress

Chronic stress can contribute to high blood pressure. Incorporate stress-reducing activities into your daily routine, such as deep breathing exercises, meditation, or spending time in nature.

Working with Your Healthcare Provider

Finally, it is crucial to maintain open communication with your healthcare provider. Share your home blood pressure readings and any concerns or questions you have. If your readings are consistently above or below your target range, your healthcare provider may need to adjust your treatment plan.

Remember, while hypertension is a severe condition, it is manageable with the right approach. By monitoring your blood pressure at home, making informed lifestyle choices, and working closely with your healthcare provider, you can take control of your health and reduce your risk of complications.

CHAPTER SEVEN

CEREBRAL VASCULAR DISEASES

"Healthy lifestyle choices are the building blocks of a vibrant life; each decision we make today shapes the strength of our tomorrow."

Stroke: A Critical Emergency We Must Address

STROKE IS ANOTHER severe cardiovascular condition that poses a significant threat to the Black Community. A stroke occurs when the blood supply to part of the brain is interrupted or reduced, depriving brain tissue of oxygen and nutrients. Within minutes, brain cells begin to die, making stroke a medical emergency that requires immediate attention. Unfortunately, strokes are more prevalent and often more severe among Black people, leading to higher rates of disability and death.

The impact of stroke on our lives can be devastating, affecting not just the individual but also families and the wider community. The risk factors for stroke are like those for other cardiovascular diseases, including hypertension, diabetes, obesity, and smoking. However, it is essential to recognize that strokes can happen to anyone, at any age, and often without warning.

Recognizing the Signs of Stroke

Time is of the essence when it comes to treating a stroke. The faster a stroke is recognized and treated, the better the chances of recovery. The acronym B.E.F.A.S.T. is a simple way to remember the most common signs of a stroke:

* Balance: sudden loss of balance, weakness, or unsteady gait

* Eyes: a sudden change in vision or vision loss in one or both eyes.

* Face drooping: One side of the face may droop or feel numb. Ask the person to smile, and check if their smile is uneven.

* Arm weakness: One arm may feel weak or numb. Ask the person to raise both arms and see if one arm drifts downward.

* Speech difficulty: The person's speech may be slurred or difficult to understand. Ask the person to repeat a simple sentence and see if they can do so clearly.

✳ Time to call 911: If someone shows any of these symptoms, even if they go away, it is crucial to contact emergency services immediately and get to the hospital as quickly as possible.

Early intervention can significantly reduce the damage caused by a stroke and improve the chances of recovery. However, despite the importance of quick action, there are often delays in seeking treatment, particularly in the Black community. This delay can result from a lack of awareness, fear, or mistrust of the healthcare system. We must educate ourselves and our loved ones about the signs of stroke and the importance of seeking immediate medical attention.

What We Can Do to Prevent Stroke

Preventing a stroke requires a proactive approach to managing the risk factors that contribute to it. For people with high blood pressure, diabetes, or a history of heart disease, it is imperative to work closely with healthcare providers to manage these conditions effectively. Regular check-ups, medication adherence, and lifestyle changes such as keeping a healthy diet, exercising regularly, and quitting smoking are all vital steps in reducing the risk of stroke.

Understanding your family history is also an essential part of stroke prevention. If strokes or other cardiovascular diseases run in your family, you may be at a higher risk. This knowledge allows you to take earlier and more aggressive steps to protect your health. Additionally, it is crucial to be aware of transient ischemic attacks (TIAs), also known as "mini strokes," which can be warning signs of a future, more severe stroke.

Empowerment Through Education and Action as the Path Forward

Strokes can be life-altering, but by empowering ourselves with knowledge and taking proactive steps, we can reduce the risk and improve outcomes if a stroke does occur. It is essential to keep the conversation going within our community about the importance of recognizing the signs of stroke, acting quickly in an emergency, and doing everything possible to prevent strokes through lifestyle changes and medical care.

Let us commit to prioritizing stroke awareness and prevention in our lives. By staying informed, encouraging regular health check-ups, and supporting each other in adopting healthier habits, we can work together to protect our community from the devastating effects of stroke. Our health is our priority, and through collective effort, we can build a future where stroke is less common and recovery is more likely.

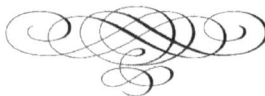

CHAPTER EIGHT

RENAL DISEASES

"Our kidneys are the silent protectors of our bodies; understanding their care is key to living a life free from the burdens of disease."

KIDNEY FAILURE, ALSO KNOWN as renal failure, is a progressive condition in which the kidneys lose their ability to function effectively, leading to the accumulation of waste products in the body. This condition can develop over time and often stems from chronic health issues like uncontrolled diabetes and hypertension.

The kidneys play a vital role in filtering the blood, removing waste, and maintaining the body's fluid and electrolyte balance. When the kidneys fail, these processes are disrupted, resulting in serious health complications. For instance, the buildup of waste in the body can lead to fluid overload, hypertension, and heart failure. Understanding the connection between kidney failure and other chronic conditions is essential in preventing further health deterioration.

Causes and Consequences of Kidney Failure

Uncontrolled diabetes can damage the blood vessels in the kidneys, leading to nephropathy, a condition that impairs kidney function. Similarly, untreated hypertension can cause the blood vessels in the kidneys to narrow, weaken, or harden, reducing their ability to filter blood effectively.

Some individuals may have a genetic predisposition to kidney disease. Understanding your family history is crucial in assessing your risk and taking preventive measures early on.

Limited access to healthcare, poor nutrition, and lack of awareness about kidney health contribute to the higher prevalence of kidney failure in the Black community. Addressing these factors through education and community outreach is vital in reducing the incidence of kidney disease.

Unhealthy lifestyle choices, such as poor diet, lack of exercise, and smoking, can worsen the risk of kidney failure. Adopting a healthier lifestyle can significantly reduce this risk.

Signs and Symptoms of Kidney Failure

* Itching

* Swelling in the feet and arms
* Difficulty breathing
* Weakness

Risk Factors for Kidney Failure

* Diabetes
* High blood pressure
* Heart disease
* Family history of kidney disease
* Obesity
* Older age
* Prolonged use of medications like ibuprofen
* Urinary tract infections

Preventive Measures

* Routine medical checkups and preventive care
* Controlling chronic conditions like diabetes and hypertension
* Eating a healthy diet low in salt, fat, and cholesterol and high in fibber
* Avoiding alcohol and exercising regularly
* Maintaining a healthy weight

* Avoiding medications that can damage the kidneys.
* Drinking plenty of clean water

The Role of Health Literacy

Health literacy is crucial in managing and preventing kidney failure. Many individuals in the Black community may not be fully aware of the signs and symptoms of kidney failure or the importance of early intervention. By increasing awareness and providing accessible information, we can empower people to take control of their health and seek timely medical care.

Hemodialysis Care

When diagnosed with end-stage renal disease (ESRD), dialysis or a kidney transplant becomes necessary to sustain life. Dialysis mimics the kidneys' function by filtering waste and excess fluids from the blood. Despite its importance, many people are hesitant to undergo dialysis, often due to a lack of understanding about the treatment or fear of the process.

Understanding Dialysis

There are two main types of dialysis hemodialysis and peritoneal dialysis. Hemodialysis involves using a machine to filter the blood outside the body, while peritoneal dialysis uses the lining of the abdomen to filter the blood internally.

Understanding these options can help patients make informed decisions about their care.

Adhering to dialysis schedules is critical for managing kidney failure. Missing dialysis sessions can lead to the buildup of toxins and fluids in the body, resulting in severe health complications such as high potassium, irregular heart rate, breathing difficulties, and generalized body fluid overload that could be life-threatening.

The process of dialysis can be physically and emotionally draining. It is essential to provide psychological support and counseling to patients undergoing dialysis to help them cope with the challenges of the treatment.

Encouraging community support and access to resources can help individuals better manage their condition. This includes information about dialysis centers, transportation options for dialysis patients, and support groups for those undergoing treatment.

The Importance of Early Detection

Early detection of kidney disease can prevent the progression to kidney failure. Regular kidney function screening, especially for high-risk patients, can lead to earlier intervention and better outcomes. Blood tests such as serum creatinine, blood urea nitrogen (BUN), and urine tests can help assess kidney function and detect problems early.

Lifestyle Modifications

Lifestyle modifications are essential for preventing kidney disease and managing existing conditions. This includes:

Reducing salt intake, limiting protein consumption, and avoiding processed foods can help protect the kidneys and manage blood pressure.

Regular physical activity helps maintain a healthy weight, control blood pressure, and improve kidney function.

Smoking can worsen kidney disease by damaging blood vessels and reducing blood flow to the kidneys. Quitting smoking is a critical step in managing kidney health.

The Wider Spectrum Beyond Kidney Failure

The health of our kidneys is critical, not only because they filter waste from the blood but also because they regulate vital functions such as electrolyte balance, blood pressure, and the production of hormones that control red blood cell production and bone health. While chronic kidney disease and kidney failure are significant concerns, it is essential not to ignore the broader spectrum of renal diseases that can affect kidney function and overall health through these ten conditions.

1. Acute Kidney Injury (AKI)

Description:

Acute Kidney Injury (AKI), previously known as acute renal failure, is a sudden and often reversible decline in kidney function. Unlike chronic kidney disease, which progresses over time, AKI occurs rapidly—sometimes within hours or days. AKI can be life-threatening, but with prompt treatment, kidney function may return to normal.

Causes:

AKI can result from a variety of factors, including severe dehydration, a drop in blood flow to the kidneys due to trauma or surgery, severe infections (sepsis), and the use of nephrotoxic drugs that can damage the kidneys. Conditions that block the urinary tract, such as kidney stones, can also lead to AKI.

Symptoms:

* Decreased urine output.

* Swelling in legs, ankles, or around the eyes

* Fatigue and confusion

* Shortness of breath

* Chest pain or pressure

Management:

Management of AKI focuses on treating the underlying cause, such as rehydrating the patient, stopping nephrotoxic drugs, and treating infections. Dialysis may be required temporarily to filter waste products from the blood until kidney function improves.

2. Glomerulonephritis

Description:

Glomerulonephritis is inflammation of the glomeruli, the tiny filtering units within the kidneys. This condition can be acute, developing suddenly, or chronic, progressing slowly. If left untreated, glomerulonephritis can lead to kidney damage and kidney failure.

Causes:

The causes of glomerulonephritis vary and can include autoimmune diseases (such as lupus), infections (like strep throat), and conditions like vasculitis (inflammation of blood vessels).

Symptoms:

 ✴ Blood in the urine (hematuria)

 ✴ Foamy urine due to excess protein (proteinuria)

 ✴ High blood pressure

 ✴ Swelling in the face, hands, feet, and abdomen

 ✴ Fatigue

Management:

Treatment depends on the cause of the inflammation. It may include medications such as corticosteroids to reduce inflammation, immunosuppressants for autoimmune causes, and antibiotics for infections. Managing blood pressure and maintaining a healthy diet are also vital treatment components.

3. Polycystic Kidney Disease (PKD)

Description:

Polycystic Kidney Disease (PKD) is a genetic disorder characterized by the growth of numerous fluid-filled cysts in the kidneys. These cysts can enlarge the kidneys and interfere with their function, leading to chronic kidney disease or kidney failure.

Causes:

PKD is caused by genetic mutations, typically inherited in an autosomal dominant or recessive pattern. This means the disease can be passed down from one or both parents.

Symptoms:

* High blood pressure
* Pain in the back or sides
* Blood in the urine
* Frequent kidney infections
* Kidney stones

Management:

While there is no cure for PKD, management focuses on treating symptoms and preventing complications. This may include controlling blood pressure, managing pain, and treating urinary tract infections promptly. In severe cases, dialysis or a kidney transplant may be necessary.

4. Nephrotic Syndrome

Description:

Nephrotic Syndrome is characterized by high protein levels in the urine, low protein levels in the blood, high cholesterol levels, and swelling. It is often the result of damage to the glomeruli and can lead to kidney failure if untreated.

Causes:

Causes of nephrotic syndrome include glomerulonephritis, diabetes, lupus, and certain types of infections. Drugs and toxins can also trigger it.

Symptoms:

Severe swelling, especially around the eyes and in the ankles and feet

* ✱ Foamy urine due to excess protein
* ✱ Weight gain due to fluid retention
* ✱ Fatigue and loss of appetite

Management:

Treatment typically involves managing the underlying cause, such as diabetes or lupus. Medications may include diuretics to reduce swelling, ACE inhibitors to control blood pressure, and statins to lower cholesterol levels. Dietary changes, such as reducing salt intake, can also be beneficial.

5. Interstitial Nephritis

Description:

Interstitial Nephritis is inflammation of the kidney's interstitial tissue, the spaces between the kidney tubules. If not treated, it can lead to acute or chronic kidney failure.

Causes:

Allergic reactions to medications, infections, and autoimmune diseases can cause interstitial nephritis. In some cases, the cause may be unknown (idiopathic).

Symptoms:

* Fever
* Rash
* Blood in the urine
* Fatigue
* Joint pain

Management:

Treatment involves finding and stopping any offending medication, treating infections, and using anti-inflammatory drugs or corticosteroids to reduce inflammation. Managing blood pressure and supporting kidney function are also critical.

6. Pyelonephritis

Description:

Pyelonephritis is a type of urinary tract infection (UTI) that has reached the kidneys. It is a severe condition that can cause permanent kidney damage if not treated promptly.

Causes:

Pyelonephritis is typically caused by bacteria that have traveled from the bladder up to the kidneys. Risk factors include frequent UTIs, urinary tract obstructions, and conditions such as diabetes.

Symptoms:

* High fever
* Back or side pain
* Nausea and vomiting
* Frequent, painful urination
* Cloudy or foul-smelling urine

Management:

Treatment usually involves antibiotics to end the infection, pain relief, and plenty of fluids to help flush the bacteria from the urinary system. In severe cases, hospitalization may be needed.

7. Renal Artery Stenosis
Description:

Renal Artery Stenosis is the narrowing of one or both arteries that supply blood to the kidneys. This condition can lead to high blood pressure (renal hypertension) and kidney damage.

Causes:

Atherosclerosis (hardening of the arteries) is the most common cause of renal artery stenosis. Another cause is fibromuscular dysplasia, which causes abnormal growth in the artery walls.

Symptoms:

* High blood pressure that is difficult to control

* Decreased kidney function.

* Fluid retention

* Swelling in the legs and feet

* Changes in urination

Management:

Treatment may include medications to control blood pressure, angioplasty to widen the narrowed artery, and lifestyle changes to manage atherosclerosis. In some cases, surgery may be necessary to bypass the blocked artery.

8. Renal Tubular Acidosis (RTA)

Description:

Renal Tubular Acidosis (RTA) is when the kidneys do not excrete acids into the urine, causing the blood to become too acidic (acidosis). RTA can lead to growth problems in children, bone disease, and kidney stones.

Causes:

RTA can be hereditary or got. It may result from chronic kidney disease, certain medications, or autoimmune disorders.

Symptoms:

* Fatigue and confusion
* Muscle weakness
* Growth retardation in children
* Bone pain or fractures
* Kidney stones

Management:

Treatment typically involves taking alkali (such as bicarbonate) to neutralize the acid in the blood, managing underlying conditions, and monitoring kidney function.

9. Kidney Stones (Nephrolithiasis)

Description:

Kidney stones are hard deposits of minerals and salts inside the kidneys. They can cause severe pain, urinary obstruction, and infections.

Causes:

Dehydration, a high-salt diet, obesity, certain genetic conditions, and metabolic disorders can cause kidney stones.

Symptoms:

* Severe pain in the back or side
* Painful urination
* Blood in the urine
* Nausea and vomiting
* Frequent urination

Management:

Small stones may pass on their own with increased fluid intake. Larger stones may require medication, lithotripsy (a procedure that uses shock waves to break up stones), or surgical removal. Preventing recurrence involves drinking plenty of fluids, dietary changes, and sometimes medications.

10. Renal Cell Carcinoma

Description:

Renal Cell Carcinoma is the most common type of kidney cancer in adults. It originates in the lining of the renal tubules and can often be successfully treated if detected early.

Causes:

Risk factors include smoking, obesity, hypertension, and certain genetic factors. It is more common in men than women and typically affects those over sixty.

Symptoms:

* Blood in the urine
* Persistent pain in the side
* Unexplained weight loss
* Fatigue
* Fever

Management:

Treatment options depend on the stage of the cancer and may include surgery to remove the tumor or kidney (nephrectomy), targeted therapy, immunotherapy, and radiation therapy. Early detection is crucial for successful treatment.

Kidney failure is a severe condition requiring vigilant management and proactive preventive measures. By understanding the causes, recognizing the symptoms, and adhering to treatment plans, we can reduce the burden of kidney disease.

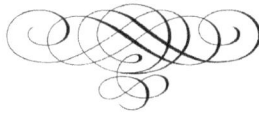

CHAPTER NINE

METABOLIC AND ENDOCRINE DISORDERS

"Mastering our body's delicate systems empowers us to prevent and manage the disorders that challenge our well-being."

DIABETES IS A SIGNIFICANT and growing concern within our community, disproportionately affecting Black people at higher rates than many other groups. This chronic condition occurs when the body cannot properly regulate blood sugar (glucose) levels, leading to health complications if not managed effectively. The prevalence of diabetes in the African community is alarming, and it underscores the importance of understanding the disease, recognizing its symptoms, and taking proactive steps to manage it.

Diabetes: A Growing Concern in the African Community

Diabetes mellitus is a chronic condition characterized by high blood glucose levels. Normal blood glucose ranges between 70 mg/dl and 100 mg/dl, serving as the body's primary energy source. Insulin, a hormone produced by the pancreas, is crucial in helping glucose enter the cells used for energy. Managing blood glucose levels becomes problematic when the pancreas malfunctions, leading to diabetes.

Black people are twice as likely as whites to develop diabetes, and they face a higher rate of hospitalization due to diabetes 2.3 times more than their white counterparts. This condition is also more prevalent in Black men than in Black women, with complications occurring more often among Black people (U.S. Department of Health and Human Services, Office of Minority Health).

There are two primary types of diabetes: Type 1 and Type 2. In Type 1 diabetes, the body produces no insulin, often due to an autoimmune disorder that develops during childhood. In Type 2 diabetes, the body either does not produce enough insulin or does not use insulin effectively, a condition that typically begins in adulthood.

Diabetes is a significant risk factor for other health complications, such as heart and kidney failure, particularly in the Black community.

It is important to remember that not managing one health problem effectively often leads to dysfunction in other body organs.

Recognizing the Symptoms of Diabetes

Diabetes can develop gradually, and in many cases, individuals may not realize they have it until they experience complications. It is essential to be aware of the common symptoms, which include:

Frequent urination: Urinating more often, especially at night.

* Excessive thirst: Feeling very thirsty despite drinking plenty of fluids.

* Increased hunger: Feeling hungry even after eating a meal.

* Unexplained weight loss: Losing weight without trying.

* Fatigue: Feeling unusually tired or weak.

* Blurred vision: Difficulty seeing clearly.

* Slow-healing sores: Cuts or sores that take a long time to heal.

* Frequent infections: Increased susceptibility to infections, particularly in the skin, gums, or bladder.

If you or someone you know is experiencing these symptoms, it is crucial to seek medical attention. Early diagnosis and intervention are vital in managing diabetes effectively and preventing complications.

Risk Factors for Diabetes

Diet: Poor dietary habits that increase blood sugar levels can worsen diabetes, primarily when the pancreas is not functioning effectively. Excess glucose is still in the blood, leading to complications. Consuming starchy and sugary foods in excess can spike blood glucose levels.

Obesity: Excess weight contributes to insulin resistance, making it difficult for body tissues to respond to insulin, thereby increasing blood glucose levels.

Stress: Stress whether physical, emotional, or physiological triggers the release of hormones like glucagon, which raises blood glucose levels. The release of cortisol during stress also makes it challenging to control blood glucose.

Age: As we age, the likelihood of developing health issues, including diabetes, increases.

Genetics: A family history of diabetes significantly raises the risk of developing the condition.

Key Strategies for Managing and Preventing Diabetes

Managing diabetes involves a combination of lifestyle changes, medication, and regular monitoring of blood sugar levels. For individuals living with diabetes, the goal is to keep blood sugar levels within a healthy range to prevent complications such as heart disease, kidney damage, nerve damage, and vision problems.

Weight Management

Being overweight is a significant risk factor for developing Type 2 diabetes. Maintaining a healthy weight (Body Mass Index, BMI of 18.5-24.9) is crucial. A BMI above 25-29 is considered overweight, and above 30 is classified as obese. Tracking your BMI can prevent overweight-related problems like uncontrolled blood glucose.

Healthy Diet

A balanced diet rich in vegetables, fruits, and whole grains is a cornerstone of diabetes management. For those with diabetes, a carbohydrate-controlled diet helps maintain normal blood glucose levels. Limiting sugar intake and consuming heart-healthy and carbohydrate-controlled foods like whole grains, vegetables, fruit, avocados, olive oil, nuts, and seeds can make a significant difference.

Regular Physical Activity

Regular physical activity helps maintain a healthy weight and manage blood glucose levels. Monitoring blood glucose before exercising is essential, as levels will likely drop during physical activity. Aim for at least 150 minutes of moderate-intensity exercise each week, such as walking or swimming. Carry a snack like an apple during exercise to address symptoms of hypoglycemia (low blood glucose), such as thirst, dizziness, and sweating.

Stress Management

Stress increases blood glucose levels and makes it difficult to control. For individuals with diabetes, stress from illness or other factors may require higher doses of diabetes medications like insulin. Managing stress is essential for controlling blood glucose.

Regular Check-ups

Health prevention and maintenance require regular check-ups, including monitoring blood glucose levels. Early detection and intervention are vital in preventing diabetes and its complications. For those already diagnosed with diabetes, it is crucial to monitor blood glucose at home, especially when taking prescription medications to manage the condition.

Preventing Complications and Living Well with Diabetes

Living with diabetes requires ongoing attention and care, but it is possible to lead a healthy and fulfilling life with the right approach. Preventing complications involves managing blood sugar levels, maintaining a healthy lifestyle, and staying informed about your condition.

Regular Check-ups: Visit your healthcare provider regularly to monitor your diabetes and address any issues early on.

Foot Care: Diabetes can reduce blood flow to the feet, increasing the risk of foot problems. Inspect your feet daily for cuts, blisters, or sores, and seek medical attention if any issues arise.

Eye Care: High blood sugar levels can damage the blood vessels in your eyes, leading to vision problems. Regular eye exams are essential to detect any changes early.

Stress Management: Stress can affect blood sugar levels, so it is essential to find healthy ways to manage stress, such as through exercise, meditation, or talking with a therapist.

By taking these steps, you can reduce your risk of complications and improve your quality of life with diabetes. It is about taking control of your health, making informed choices, and working closely with your healthcare team to manage your condition effectively.

Medications and Insulin Management

Managing diabetes effectively often requires more than just lifestyle changes; for many, medications and insulin therapy play a crucial role in keeping blood sugar levels within a healthy range.

Oral Medications for Type 2 Diabetes

Oral diabetes medications may include metformin, Actos, and Prandin. The medical management approach may vary from person to person, depending on factors such as health history and other comorbidities. With Type 2 diabetes, oral medications are often prescribed to help control blood sugar levels. These medications work in different ways, including:

Stimulating insulin production: Medications like sulfonylureas (e.g., glipizide, glyburide) help the pancreas produce more insulin.

Improving insulin sensitivity: Drugs such as metformin improve the body's sensitivity to insulin, making it easier for glucose to enter the cells.

Reducing glucose production: Some medications, like metformin, also decrease the amount of glucose the liver produces.

Slowing carbohydrate absorption: Medications like alpha-glucosidase inhibitors slow down carbohydrates' absorption in the digestive tract, which helps prevent blood sugar spikes after meals.

Each medication works differently, and it is essential to follow your healthcare provider's instructions carefully to ensure the best results. Regular monitoring of blood sugar levels is crucial to determine how well your medication is working and whether adjustments are needed.

Insulin Therapy

Insulin comes in various forms, including short-acting, intermediate-acting, and long-acting, defined by how quickly it starts working when it peaks and how long it lasts in the body. Insulin can be administered through needles, vials, pens, or insulin pumps. One of the most prominent side effects of diabetes medications, especially insulin, is hypoglycemia, which is why monitoring blood glucose before taking these medications is essential. Your doctor will guide you on when to hold or take your medication based on your blood glucose levels.

For those with Type 1 diabetes or advanced Type 2 diabetes, insulin therapy is often necessary to manage blood sugar levels. Insulin is a hormone that helps glucose enter the cells, and without it, blood sugar levels can become critically high.

There are several types of insulin, including:

* Rapid-acting insulin: Works quickly to reduce blood sugar levels after meals (e.g., insulin lispro, insulin aspart).

* Short-acting insulin: It takes longer to work than rapid-acting insulin but is still used before meals (e.g., regular insulin).

* Intermediate-acting insulin provides longer-lasting blood sugar control and is often combined with short or rapid-acting insulin (e.g., NPH insulin).

* Long-acting insulin: Provides a steady release of insulin over 24 hours or more, helping to control blood sugar levels between meals and overnight (e.g., insulin glargine, insulin detemir).

Best Practices for Insulin Management

Managing insulin therapy requires careful attention to detail. Here are some best practices to keep in mind:

* Monitor blood sugar levels regularly:

Check your blood sugar levels as your healthcare provider recommends, especially before meals and bedtime. This will help you determine how much insulin you need and when you need it.

✴ Use the correct dosage:

Always use the insulin dosage prescribed by your healthcare provider. Using too much or too little insulin can lead to hypoglycemia (low blood sugar) or hyperglycemia (high blood sugar), both of which can lead to critical situations.

✴ Store insulin properly.

Insulin should be stored in a cool, dry place. It is essential to check the expiration date before use. Insulin that has been exposed to extreme temperatures or has expired may not work as effectively.

✴ Rotate injection sites.

To prevent skin irritation and ensure even insulin absorption, rotate the sites where you inject insulin. Common injection sites include the abdomen, thighs, and upper arms (Subcutaneous tissues).

✴ Be prepared for emergencies.

Carry a quick source of glucose, such as glucose tablets or a snack, in case of low blood sugar. It is also a good idea to wear a medical alert bracelet that identifies you as someone with diabetes.

The Role of Healthcare Providers

Working closely with your healthcare provider is crucial in managing diabetes, especially regarding medications and insulin therapy. Regular check-ups allow adjustments to your treatment plan as needed, and your provider can offer guidance on handling any challenges.

Remember, diabetes management is a dynamic process that requires ongoing attention and care. By staying informed, following your treatment plan, and maintaining open communication with your healthcare team, you can effectively manage your diabetes and reduce the risk of complications.

Preventing Complications and Living Well with Diabetes

Managing diabetes is a continuous process beyond simply controlling blood glucose levels. It involves taking proactive steps to prevent complications and maintain a fulfilling, healthy life. I want to share some advanced insights, community-focused approaches, and practical advice to help you integrate diabetes management into your daily life.

The Ripple Effect of Diabetes Management

In previous chapters, we have discussed the importance of monitoring blood glucose and maintaining a healthy lifestyle. Now, let us explore how these actions have a ripple effect, influencing physical health and emotional and social well-being. For example, consistent management of diabetes not only reduces the risk of complications like heart disease and neuropathy but contributes to mental clarity, energy levels, and overall quality of life.

Imagine a scenario where someone in our community, let us call her Maria, neglects her diabetes management due to a lack of time and support. Over the years, she starts experiencing symptoms of neuropathy, leading to constant pain and difficulty walking. This affects her ability to work, socialize, and enjoy her hobbies, impacting her mental health. This is a stark reminder that effective diabetes management is not just about preventing physical complications but about preserving the ability to live life to the fullest.

Embrace Technology and Personalized Medicine

In today's world, technology offers new avenues for managing diabetes more effectively. Continuous glucose monitors (CGMs) and insulin pumps provide real-time data and automation, making stable blood glucose levels more manageable. These tools are becoming increasingly accessible and can be a game-changer, particularly for those who struggle with traditional management methods.

Moreover, personalized medicine is advancing rapidly, offering treatments tailored to an individual's genetic makeup, lifestyle, and specific health conditions. For instance, pharmacogenomics, the study of how genes affect a person's response to drugs, is beginning to play a role in selecting the most effective diabetes medications for each person. By embracing these innovations, we can move towards a future where diabetes management is more precise and personalized.

Building a Supportive Community

While individual efforts are essential, managing diabetes is also a community endeavor. Support from family, friends, and community organizations can significantly affect your ability to manage diabetes effectively. For example, local health initiatives that provide access to affordable healthy foods, exercise programs, and diabetes education can substantially affect health outcomes.

Consider organizing or joining a support group in your area. These groups can offer practical advice, emotional support, and a sense of camaraderie that makes managing diabetes less isolated. Community health workers and local clinics can also provide resources and guidance tailored to the specific needs of our community.

Q&A: Addressing Common Concerns

Q: What should I do if I feel overwhelmed by my diabetes management routine?

A: It is expected to feel overwhelmed at times. Start by breaking down your routine into smaller, manageable steps.

Prioritize the most critical aspects, such as taking your medications and monitoring your blood glucose. Seek support from your healthcare team and loved ones, and do not hesitate to ask for help when needed.

Q: How can I stay motivated to maintain a healthy lifestyle?

A: Motivation can fluctuate, but setting realistic goals and celebrating small victories can help. Surround yourself with supportive people who encourage your efforts. Remember that each healthy choice is an investment in your future well-being.

Q: What role does stress play in managing diabetes?

A: Stress can significantly affect blood glucose levels, making diabetes management more challenging. Incorporating stress management techniques, such as mindfulness, regular exercise, and relaxation exercises, into your routine can help mitigate these effects.

Personalized Advice for Living Well with Diabetes

As we move forward, let us remember that living well with diabetes is a journey that requires both knowledge and action. Reflect on the strategies and insights we have discussed so far, and think about how you can apply them to your own life. Whether incorporating regular physical activity, making dietary adjustments, or leveraging new technologies, every step brings you closer to a healthier, more empowered life.

Managing diabetes is not just about preventing complications—it is about thriving. It is about maintaining independence, enjoying your hobbies, and staying connected with the people you love. By taking an active role in your health and seeking support when needed, you can live a whole, vibrant life despite the challenges of diabetes.

Obesity

The impact of obesity on diabetes management cannot be underestimated. Obesity makes body tissues less sensitive to insulin, making it more challenging to control blood glucose levels as body weight increases.

Personalized Strategies for Managing Obesity

Obesity goes beyond knowing the medical definitions and statistics it is about recognizing how it impacts our lives and what we can do to take control. Obesity is a complex issue, influenced by various factors, including our environment, culture, and personal habits. Let us explore how we can tackle it together, focusing on practical, personalized strategies that fit into our daily lives.

Embracing a Balanced Diet with Small Changes for Big Impact

When it comes to dieting, small, consistent changes can lead to significant results. Start by assessing your current eating habits. Are you consuming too many processed foods or sugary drinks? If so, consider swapping out one unhealthy item for a healthier choice each week. For example, replace sugary sodas with water or herbal tea, or choose a whole fruit instead of a sweet snack.

Meal planning can also play a crucial role in managing weight. Preparing meals at home gives you control over what goes into your food, allowing you to make healthier choices. If time is a constraint, batch cooking on weekends or prepping ingredients in advance can make it easier to stick to a balanced diet during the week.

Incorporating Physical Activity by Making It Fun and Routine

Physical activity does not have to be a chore—it can be something you enjoy. Think about activities that make you feel good and fit into your lifestyle. Whether dancing, walking, or joining a local sports team, the key is finding something you look forward to doing. Start small if you are new to exercise, and gradually increase the intensity and duration as you build your fitness level.

To make physical activity a routine, try setting aside specific times each day for movement. Even 10 to 15 minutes of exercise can make a difference. Remember, the goal is to find what works for you and to stay consistent.

Addressing Emotional Eating with Mindfulness and Support

Emotional eating is a common challenge, often triggered by stress, boredom, or negative emotions. To manage this, practice mindfulness pay attention to what you are eating, how much you are eating, and why you are eating. Ask yourself, "Am I famished or eating out of habit or emotion?"

Seeking support from friends, family, or a counselor can also be helpful. Sometimes, just talking about what is going on in your life can alleviate the emotional triggers that lead to overeating. Consider keeping a journal to track your emotions and eating patterns, which can help you find triggers and develop healthier coping mechanisms.

You are Not Alone; Leverage Community Resources

Managing obesity is challenging, but you must not do it alone. Look for community resources that can support your journey. This could be a local weight management group, a fitness program at your community center, or online support groups where you can share experiences and tips with others facing similar challenges.

If you struggle to access healthy food or safe places to exercise, consider contacting local organizations that help. Many communities have programs that provide fresh produce at discounted rates or free fitness classes. These resources are there to help you succeed, so do not hesitate to use them.

Celebrate Progress, Not Perfection, To Set Realistic Goals

Finally, managing obesity is a journey, not a destination. Set realistic, achievable goals for yourself, and celebrate your progress. Whether losing a few pounds, improving your stamina, or simply feeling more energetic, every step forward is a victory.

It is essential to focus on progress, not perfection. There will be setbacks, but that's part of the process. What matters is that you keep moving forward, learning from each experience, and staying committed to your health.

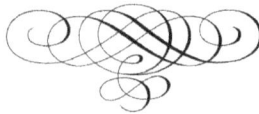

CHAPTER TEN

CHRONIC AND INFECTIOUS DISEASES

"Addressing chronic and infectious diseases requires a commitment to prevention, education, and equitable access to care, ensuring every community can thrive in health and well-being."

CHRONIC AND INFECTIOUS diseases are complex health conditions that significantly affect individuals and communities. A comprehensive understanding of these diseases is crucial for effective prevention and management. Chronic diseases, such as asthma, diabetes, and heart disease, are long-term conditions that typically progress slowly and can be managed but not cured. They often require ongoing medical attention and lifestyle management. Infectious diseases, on the other hand, are caused by pathogens and can spread from person to person or through other means like contaminated food, water, or insect bites.

Unlike chronic diseases, many infectious diseases can be prevented, treated, or even cured with appropriate measures like vaccinations, medications, and public health interventions. Both types of diseases pose significant challenges, particularly in communities with limited healthcare and health education access. Effective management and prevention of chronic and infectious diseases are essential for improving public health outcomes and reducing healthcare access and quality disparities. In this chapter, we will examine four of these.

Asthma

Asthma is a chronic respiratory condition characterized by inflammation and narrowing of the airways, making breathing difficult. It affects people of all ages but often begins in childhood. Among the Black community, asthma is rampant, with higher rates and more severe outcomes compared to other populations.

Managing asthma requires a holistic approach to healthcare. It's not just about addressing the medical aspects of the disease, but also the broader social determinants that impact health. A combination of environmental exposures, access to healthcare, and socio-economic factors influences the disparity in asthma rates among different populations. These underlying issues often compound the challenges individuals face in managing asthma.

Asthma symptoms can vary in severity but include shortness of breath, chest tightness or pain, wheezing a whistling sound when breathing and persistent coughing, particularly at night or early in the morning.

These indicators can be triggered by various factors such as allergens like pollen, mold, and pet dander; air pollutants including smoke and chemicals; respiratory infections; physical activity; and even stress or strong emotions. For many, exposure to these triggers is more common due to living in environments with higher levels of pollution or allergens, further worsening the severity of asthma symptoms.

Managing asthma effectively involves avoiding known triggers and using medications to control symptoms. Individuals with asthma should work closely with their healthcare providers to create an asthma action plan that includes daily management strategies and specific steps to take during an asthma attack. Medications for asthma typically include inhaled corticosteroids, which reduce inflammation and mucus production in the airways, and bronchodilators, which help to open the airways by relaxing the muscles around them. These medications are essential for controlling symptoms and preventing asthma attacks.

Addressing asthma also requires tackling the environmental and social factors that worsen the condition. Improving air quality in living environments, reducing exposure to allergens, and ensuring consistent access to medical care are critical components of effective asthma management.

Education also plays a key role; learning how to use inhalers correctly, recognizing early signs of an asthma attack, and knowing when to seek medical help can significantly improve outcomes. Preventive care and ongoing education about asthma are vital in reducing the frequency and severity of attacks and enhancing the quality of life for those affected.

Liver Cirrhosis

Liver cirrhosis is a chronic and progressive disease that results in the scarring (fibrosis) of liver tissue, leading to impaired liver function. This condition often develops over many years due to long-term damage from various causes, such as chronic hepatitis B and C infections, excessive alcohol consumption, or non-alcoholic fatty liver disease (NAFLD). Within the Black community, liver cirrhosis has become an increasing concern, with rates of liver disease rising due to a combination of genetic predisposition, lifestyle factors, and limited access to healthcare.

The symptoms of liver cirrhosis can vary, but they often include fatigue, weakness, loss of appetite, weight loss, jaundice (yellowing of the skin and eyes), swelling in the legs and abdomen (ascites), itching, easy bruising or bleeding, and cognitive changes such as confusion (hepatic encephalopathy).

These symptoms typically appear as the liver becomes increasingly unable to perform its vital functions, including detoxifying the blood, producing essential proteins, and regulating various bodily processes. For many in the Black community, these symptoms may be overlooked or misattributed to other causes, leading to delays in diagnosis and treatment.

Liver cirrhosis is mainly caused by chronic hepatitis B and C infections, prolonged heavy alcohol use, non-alcoholic fatty liver disease, and inherited liver disorders such as hemochromatosis or Wilson's disease. In the Black community, the prevalence of risk factors like obesity, diabetes, and hypertension further increases the likelihood of developing liver cirrhosis. Addressing these underlying conditions through lifestyle changes, such as adopting a healthier diet, reducing alcohol consumption, and managing chronic diseases effectively, can help prevent or slow the progression of cirrhosis.

While liver cirrhosis is a severe and potentially life-threatening condition, its progression can often be managed with proper medical care and lifestyle modifications. Treatment may include medications to manage symptoms or complications, regular monitoring of liver function, and, in severe cases, consideration for liver transplantation.

Increasing awareness of liver cirrhosis, its risk factors, and the importance of early intervention is essential. Preventive measures, such as vaccinations for hepatitis B, regular screenings for liver disease, and education on the dangers of excessive alcohol use, can significantly reduce the incidence of liver cirrhosis and improve overall health outcomes.

Sexually Transmitted Diseases (STDs)

Sexually Transmitted Diseases (STDs) encompass a range of infections transmitted primarily through sexual contact, including chlamydia, gonorrhea, syphilis, HIV, and herpes. These diseases represent a significant public health challenge within the Black community, where infection rates are disproportionately higher compared to other populations. This disparity is driven by a variety of factors, including limited access to healthcare, social stigma, economic challenges, and systemic inequalities that affect health behaviors and outcomes.

Chlamydia and gonorrhea, two of the most common STDs, often present with symptoms such as pain during urination, abnormal genital discharge, and, in women, pelvic pain. However, many individuals with these infections may be asymptomatic, leading to undiagnosed and untreated cases that can result in serious complications, such as infertility or chronic pelvic pain. Syphilis, another serious STD, progresses through stages, starting with sores at the site of infection and potentially leading to severe systemic symptoms if left untreated. HIV, the virus that causes AIDS, initially presents with flu-like symptoms before entering a prolonged asymptomatic phase. Without treatment, HIV weakens the immune system, leaving the body vulnerable to opportunistic infections and cancers. Herpes, characterized by painful blisters or sores, can cause recurrent outbreaks and has no cure, although antiviral medications can help manage symptoms.

Preventing and managing STDs requires a comprehensive approach that includes accessible testing and treatment, addressing social and cultural factors, and promoting safe sexual practices like condom use, regular testing, and vaccinations such as HPV and hepatitis B to prevent certain STDs and complications.

For those diagnosed with STD, prompt treatment is vital to prevent complications and reduce the risk of transmitting the infection to others. Antibiotics are effective for bacterial STDs like chlamydia, gonorrhea, and syphilis, while antiviral medications are used to manage viral infections like HIV and herpes. It is also important to foster open communication about sexual health and reduce the stigma associated with STDs, which can deter individuals from seeking necessary care. Community outreach and culturally sensitive healthcare services can play a significant role in encouraging prevention and treatment, reducing the burden of STDs in our community.

Malaria

Malaria is a life-threatening disease caused by Plasmodium parasites, transmitted to humans through the bites of infected female Anopheles mosquitoes. While malaria is not common in the United States, it remains a significant health issue in many African countries where the disease is endemic. Malaria disproportionately affects people, particularly in Africa, where it is a leading cause of illness and death, especially among young children and pregnant women.

The symptoms of malaria typically include high fever, chills, sweating, headache, nausea, vomiting, muscle pain, fatigue, and anemia. These symptoms often appear within 10-15 days after a mosquito bite and can be severe, leading to complications such as cerebral malaria, organ failure, and death if not treated promptly. The impact of malaria is not just limited to the individual; it also has profound social and economic consequences for affected communities, contributing to cycles of poverty and limiting access to education and economic opportunities.

One of the most effective preventive measures is using insecticide-treated bed nets, which protect against mosquito bites during sleep. These nets are a simple yet powerful tool in reducing malaria transmission. Additionally, taking antimalarial medications, particularly for travelers to high-risk areas, can prevent disease development. Public health efforts to eliminate standing water, where mosquitoes breed, are also crucial in reducing the mosquito population and the spread of malaria.

For those who contract malaria, prompt and suitable treatment is essential to prevent severe illness and death. Antimalarial drugs, such as artemisinin-based combination therapies (ACTs), are the most effective treatment for malaria. These medications kill the parasite in the bloodstream and prevent its replication. However, access to these treatments can be limited in some areas, highlighting the need for continued global efforts to improve healthcare infrastructure and ensure that effective malaria treatment is available to all who need it.

It is crucial for those living in or traveling to malaria-endemic regions to be aware of the risks and take proper preventive measures. In the broader fight against malaria, supporting global initiatives that aim to reduce the incidence of the disease through prevention, treatment, and research is essential in moving towards the goal of malaria eradication.

Conclusion

Chronic and infectious diseases are not just medical issues they reflect how well we prioritize and manage our health. As we have learned in this chapter, identifying the risks, staying vigilant with preventive practices, and seeking timely medical care are crucial steps in reducing the burden of these diseases.

Education and awareness are our strongest allies in this fight. By educating ourselves and our communities about the importance of regular check-ups, safe practices, and early interventions, we empower each other to take control of our health.

Remember: our community's strength lies in its individuals' health. Let us commit to making informed decisions, supporting one another, and fostering an environment where health is a shared responsibility.

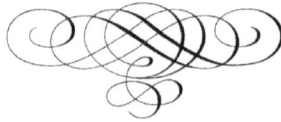

CHAPTER ELEVEN

CANCER

"Early detection and proactive care are our most powerful tools in the fight against cancer, especially when we stand together as the Black community, supporting each other through every step."

CANCER IS ONE OF the most challenging health issues affecting humankind worldwide, and its impact is concerning to me and worth learning and teaching about. The frequency of certain cancers among our race is higher than in other racial groups, which underscores the need for targeted education, early detection, and comprehensive care strategies.

Figuring out the types of cancers that are most common in the Black population, along with the importance of early detection and the benefits of lifestyle changes, can help reduce the incidence and mortality rates associated with this disease. Let us dig deeper.

Common Cancers in the Black Population

Among these are prostate cancer, breast cancer, colorectal cancer, and lung cancer. Prostate cancer, for example, is more common and more aggressive in Black men than in men of other races. Breast cancer, while less common in Black women compared to white women, tends to be diagnosed at a later stage, making it more challenging to treat. Colorectal cancer also presents a significant risk, with higher mortality rates seen in the Black community due to later diagnoses and disparities in access to care.

Genetic factors, environmental exposures, and lifestyle choices contribute to the higher incidence rates, but access to healthcare and socioeconomic factors also play critical roles. This is why early detection and regular screenings are paramount as the first step.

Importance of Early Detection and Regular Screenings

Early detection is one of the most effective strategies in the fight against cancer. When cancer is caught in its initial stages, treatment is more likely to be successful, and the chances of survival increase significantly.

Fortunately, many cancers are diagnosed at later stages when the disease is more advanced and more challenging to treat. This delay in diagnosis is often due to a lack of access to regular screenings, mistrust of the healthcare system, and a lack of awareness about the importance of early detection.

Regular screenings such as mammograms for breast cancer, prostate-specific antigen (PSA) tests for prostate cancer, and colonoscopies for colorectal cancer are crucial. These tests can identify cancerous changes before symptoms appear, allowing for timely intervention.

It is essential to stay informed about the recommended screening schedules and make these tests a regular part of our healthcare routine. Additionally, genetic testing can be a valuable tool for those with a family history of cancer, providing information that can guide preventive measures and early intervention strategies.

Treatment and Management Strategies for Different Types of Cancer

The treatment and management of cancer vary depending on the type and stage of the disease and the patient's overall health. For most cancers, treatment options include surgery, radiation therapy, chemotherapy, immunotherapy, and targeted therapy. The choice of treatment is often guided by the specific characteristics of the cancer, such as its size, location, and whether it has spread to other parts of the body.

Access to quality healthcare can impact the availability and effectiveness of cancer treatment. Financial constraints, lack of insurance, and geographic barriers can limit access to state-of-the-art therapies and experienced oncologists. It is crucial to address these disparities by advocating for equitable access to healthcare services and ensuring that all individuals, regardless of race or socioeconomic status, receive the care they need.

Managing cancer also involves addressing the physical, emotional, and social challenges that come with the disease. Patients and their families need comprehensive support systems that include medical care, psychological counseling, nutritional support, and assistance navigating the healthcare system. The journey through cancer treatment can be overwhelming, but with the proper support, patients can manage their treatment and maintain their quality of life.

Lifestyle Changes to Reduce Cancer Risk

While some risk factors for cancer, such as genetics, cannot be changed, many lifestyle factors can be modified to reduce the risk of developing cancer. Diet, physical activity, smoking, and alcohol consumption are all areas where individuals can make changes that significantly impact their cancer risk.

A diet rich in fruits, vegetables, whole grains, and lean proteins can help reduce cancer risk. Limiting the intake of processed foods, red meats, and foods high in fat and sugar is also beneficial. Regular physical activity helps maintain a healthy weight, which is important because obesity is a known risk factor for several types of cancer, including breast and colorectal cancers.

Smoking is one of the most significant risk factors for cancer, particularly lung cancer. Quitting smoking at any age can reduce the risk of developing cancer and improve overall health. Similarly, reducing alcohol consumption can lower the risk of cancers such as breast, liver, and esophageal cancer.

Protecting the skin from excessive sun exposure, a risk factor for skin cancer, is also essential. Using sunscreen, wearing protective clothing, and avoiding tanning beds are simple yet effective measures that can help prevent skin cancer.

Support Systems and Resources for Cancer Patients and Survivors

Cancer affects the patient, their family, friends, and the community. Support systems are essential for helping patients navigate the challenges of cancer treatment and recovery. Emotional support from family and friends can provide the strength and motivation needed to endure the rigors of treatment. Support groups, both in-person and online, offer a space for patients and survivors to share their experiences, learn from others, and gain emotional and practical support.

Together with emotional support, practical resources are vital for cancer patients. These include access to financial assistance programs, transportation services for medical appointments, and educational resources about the disease and its treatment. Healthcare providers play a key role in connecting patients with these resources and helping them manage the logistical aspects of cancer care.

Survivorship care is another critical component of cancer treatment. After completing treatment, cancer survivors need ongoing care to monitor for recurrence and manage any long-term side effects of treatment. This care should include regular follow-up visits with healthcare providers and support for emotional and mental health. Survivorship programs that address the unique needs of cancer survivors can help individuals transition from active treatment to a new normal, with a focus on maintaining health and well-being.

Conclusion

Cancer is a global health crisis, with over nineteen million new cases diagnosed each year and nearly ten million deaths worldwide, according to the World Health Organization (WHO). The impact of this disease is profound, affecting individuals, families, and entire communities. In the Black race, cancer presents unique challenges due to disparities in access to healthcare, later-stage diagnoses, and higher mortality rates. However, these challenges are not insurmountable.

Studies have shown that when cancer is detected at an early stage, the five-year survival rate can be as high as 90%, compared to just 10% for cancers diagnosed at later stages. This underscores the importance of regular screenings and awareness programs that target high-risk populations, including Black communities where cancers like prostate, breast, and colorectal are particularly prevalent.

Globally, lifestyle factors such as smoking, poor diet, physical inactivity, and alcohol consumption contribute to nearly 30% of cancer deaths. By making informed lifestyle changes quitting smoking, reducing alcohol intake, maintaining a healthy diet, and engaging in regular physical activity we can significantly reduce the risk of developing cancer. The WHO estimates these lifestyle modifications could prevent up to 50% of cancers.

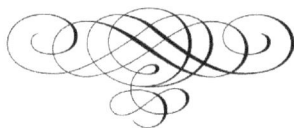

PART FOUR

TAKING ACTION

CHAPTER TWELVE

FAMILY HEALTH HISTORY

"Our past carries the keys to our future health—knowing our family's history can unlock the power of prevention."

Importance of Knowing Family Health History

FAMILY HEALTH HISTORY plays a significant role in shaping our approach to personal and community health. Some diseases are genetic or run through a family lineage, making it essential for individuals to understand the health challenges faced by their ancestors. For example, conditions like cancer, heart failure, and diabetes often affect multiple generations. Recognizing that your grandparents and parents had the same disorder can serve as a critical wake-up call, urging the next generation to take proactive measures to prevent the reoccurrence of these diseases.

Therefore, understanding one's family health history is essential to preventive healthcare. Chronic diseases such as diabetes, heart disease, hypertension, and certain cancers are mainly known to run in families, which makes tracking this history a powerful tool for anticipating potential health risks. When we know the illnesses that have affected our close relatives, we are better equipped to make informed decisions regarding our health. This knowledge allows us to take preventive actions before these conditions become more severe, reducing the likelihood of long-term complications or early mortality.

In many communities, especially among Black families, the idea of tracing family health history may seem unfamiliar or not prioritized. Family health conversations are often not as daily as about other life issues. However, understanding family health patterns offers an invaluable opportunity to take control of our health outcomes. Your health story is partly written in the experiences of your parents, grandparents, and other family members.

By identifying patterns and shared risk factors, we can work toward early detection and prevention of diseases that disproportionately affect our community. Diseases such as hypertension, heart disease, and certain cancers have been shown to impact Black communities at higher rates than others. Knowing the genetic risks within your family empowers you to confront those risks head-on, enabling you to take steps that protect your health and future generations.

For example, if multiple family members have been diagnosed with diabetes, this knowledge creates an opportunity for you to act pre-emptively. Understanding the genetic predisposition allows individuals to make more informed lifestyle changes, such as adopting a balanced diet and regular exercise to prevent or delay the onset of the disease. In this way, the potential impact of family health history extends beyond the individual, offering a path toward improving the overall health of an entire family. Knowing your family history transforms what could seem like an inevitable health outcome into actionable insights that can alter the course of your life and future generations.

Health is not just a matter of chance. It combines environmental factors, lifestyle choices, and the knowledge we gain from our family health history. This proactive approach enables us to become more vigilant about our health choices, seeking regular checkups, making healthy dietary changes, exercising regularly, and monitoring our mental and emotional well-being.

With these tools, individuals and families are better prepared to take charge of their health and well-being. Through informed action, we can improve individual and collective outcomes by closing the gap on preventable diseases. The health of an entire community can shift when families are equipped with knowledge, empowered to make better health choices, and encouraged to pass down this information to future generations.

Family health history often allows us to take actions we might not have otherwise considered. If, for instance, your parent or grandparent suffered from heart disease or hypertension, understanding their medical history enables you to discuss your risk factors with your healthcare provider more proactively. Your physician may recommend preventive measures such as early screening for heart conditions, adopting a heart-healthy diet, or making specific lifestyle changes to reduce your risks.

Taking control of our family history is a responsibility and a form of empowerment. In doing so, we can bridge the gaps between generations, ensuring that the health challenges of the past do not have to define the future.

By gaining insight into the conditions that have affected our family members, we can take preventive steps, manage existing conditions more effectively, and work together toward a healthier, more informed community. The family health history is not just a medical record; it is a tool for change, allowing us to rewrite our health outcomes and create a legacy of wellness for those who come after us.

How it Helps in Making Informed Health Decisions.

Understanding your family health history goes beyond knowing the illnesses affecting your relatives. It is a powerful tool in shaping your health, decisions, and well-being. For the Black community, where genetic predispositions and socio-economic factors often compound health risks, knowing your family's medical background becomes even more crucial. Here are the five most critical benefits of knowing your family health history and how it can be a driving force in making informed health decisions for you and future generations.

Early Detection and Prevention

Knowing your family health history allows for the early detection of potential health risks. When you are aware of diseases that have affected your family, such as diabetes, hypertension, or heart disease, you can take proactive measures to prevent them. This might include lifestyle changes, regular screenings, or discussions with your doctor about preventative treatments. For example, knowing about a family history of heart disease might lead you to monitor your blood pressure closely or adopt a heart-healthy diet.

Personalized Medical Care

Family health history provides valuable information that helps doctors tailor medical care to your needs. Rather than following generalized recommendations, your healthcare provider can suggest targeted screenings or treatments based on your inherited risks. This personalized approach is fundamental within the Black community, where some conditions like hypertension may require earlier or more specialized interventions.

Informed Decision-Making

With knowledge of your family health background, you can make more informed decisions about your healthcare. This information lets you weigh your risks, consult with healthcare professionals, and decide on lifestyle changes or treatments that best suit your needs. Whether deciding to undergo genetic testing, opting for regular screenings, or choosing specific preventive measures, a well-documented family history can guide you in making these important health decisions.

Encourages Family Conversations

Sharing your family health history fosters open discussions within the family about inherited risks. This encourages family members to take health seriously and promotes collective action towards wellness. When families openly discuss health risks, they can work together to adopt healthier habits and support one another in taking proactive steps, such as eating healthier or exercising regularly.

Improved Health Outcomes for Future Generations

Understanding family health history benefits you and future generations. By documenting and sharing health information, you help children and grandchildren be better equipped to manage inherited risks. This knowledge empowers them to make early, informed decisions, increasing their chances of preventing or managing diseases that may run in the family.

The experiences of our loved ones provide a unique perspective when making health-related decisions. When you can relate to the choices and outcomes faced by family members, it becomes easier to grasp medical management options and the course of care. This insight allows you to approach your health proactively, with the added benefit of personal history guiding your understanding and decisions. Through this connection to the past, Black people can make more informed, confident choices for their future well-being.

How to Gather and Record Family Health Information.

Gathering and recording family health information is essential to taking proactive control of your health. However, for many, this process can feel overwhelming, mainly if health issues have rarely been discussed within the family. The Black community may face unique challenges when it comes to discussing health openly due to cultural stigmas or historical mistrust of medical systems. Despite these barriers, it is crucial to understand that knowing your family health history can empower you to make informed choices and promote a healthier future for yourself and your loved ones.

The first step in gathering family health information is to engage in open and compassionate conversations with relatives. It is essential to approach these discussions sensitively, as health can be a delicate topic for some. Start by speaking to older relatives, who often hold valuable insights into family medical history.

Ask about any known conditions such as heart disease, diabetes, cancer, hypertension, or other chronic illnesses that might run in the family. In addition, ask about lifestyle factors, such as dietary habits or exercise routines, which could have influenced health outcomes over time. Remember to record the age of onset for any conditions, as this information can help doctors identify potential risk factors more accurately.

Once you have gathered this information, recording it clearly and organizing it is essential. Keeping a written record or creating a digital file is a great way to ensure the data is accessible whenever needed. Be sure to include as many details as possible, including the types of conditions, their severity, and any treatments that have been used. Over time, this record can be updated as more information becomes available or as family members experience new health developments.

Sharing this information with healthcare providers is the final step in utilizing family health history to make informed health decisions. If necessary, your doctor can use this knowledge to recommend preventive screenings, lifestyle adjustments, or genetic counseling. The more your healthcare provider knows about your family's health, the better they can personalize your care plan.

Template for Gathering and Recording Family Health Information

Step 1: Start with Your Immediate Family

Begin by collecting health information from your closest family members: parents, siblings, children, and grandparents. This forms the foundation of your family's health history.

Relation:

Age:

Current Health Status:

Known Medical Conditions:

Age at Diagnosis (if applicable):

Cause of Death (if deceased):

Lifestyle Factors (smoking, alcohol use, exercise habits, etc.):

Repeat this process for each immediate family member and any other extended family members, such as aunts and uncles, who may be affected by any concerning or hereditary chronic issues.

Step 2: Document Lifestyle and Environmental Factors

Alongside medical history, it is essential to note lifestyle and environmental factors that may influence health. These can be just as important in understanding the risk of developing certain diseases.

Dietary Habits (typical family diet):

Physical Activity (exercise frequency and type):

Substance Use (alcohol, smoking, drug use):

Environmental Exposures (living conditions, pollution, etc.):

Work-Related Health Risks (exposure to harmful substances, stress levels):

Step 3: Use Health-Tracking Tools or Apps

To simplify the process, consider using health-tracking tools or apps to document and organize your family's health information in one place.

Name of App/Tool:

Information to Record (conditions, treatments, family health notes):

Frequency of Updates (weekly, monthly, annually):

Step 4: Keep Information Updated

It is important to update this information regularly as family members age or new conditions emerge. Track annual check-ups, new diagnoses, and lifestyle changes.

Date of Last Update:

Changes Noted:

Step 5: Share the Information with Healthcare Providers

Once you have a well-documented family health history, please share it with your healthcare provider. This will help them provide personalized care, identify potential risks, and suggest preventive measures.

Healthcare Provider Name:

Date Information Shared:

Key Risk Factors Identified by Provider:

Recommended Preventive Actions:

I have created a tabulated template as an example to help you organize your family health information. It includes sections for immediate and extended family members, lifestyle factors, tools for tracking health, and more.

Family Member	Relationship	Health Conditions	Age at Diagnosis	Lifestyle Factors (Diet, Exercise, Smoking)	Medications/ Treatment	Outcome (Recovery, Complications)
Parent 1 (e.g., Father)						
Parent 2 (e.g., Mother)						
Sibling one						
Grandparent one						
Grandparent two						

Additional Tools for Tracking Health Information

Health Tracking Apps: Apps like MyFitnessPal, Apple Health, or Google Fit can be used to track family health patterns and lifestyle habits.

Medical Records: Keep copies of medical records or lab results for family members to monitor and share with healthcare providers.

Family Health Tree: Create a visual family health tree that shows patterns of diseases across generations.

This table can be expanded or customized based on your family history needs. The goal is to capture detailed and actionable information. After seeing a doctor, you must conduct open discussions with parents and family members, including grandparents and siblings, about medical diagnoses.

One thing I have noticed is that most Black parents do not openly discuss specific health issues. Some may want to keep the pain, suffering, and stress away from their children without knowing the significance of open conversion in disease prevention and health maintenance.

Using Family History to Anticipate

Understanding your family health history is critical in anticipating potential health issues. By identifying patterns of diseases that affect multiple generations, we can take proactive steps to mitigate risks. For example, if there is a history of heart disease or diabetes in your family, you are already armed with the knowledge that these conditions could affect you or your children. This allows for timely interventions, such as lifestyle modifications, regular screenings, and discussions with healthcare providers.

Knowing your family history helps in disease prevention and health maintenance. For instance, if you know that your grandfather had heart failure, your father also had heart disease, and one of your siblings is already affected, this is a red flag for the next generation.

The knowledge of this family pattern should prompt you and your family members to begin taking proactive steps such as:

Yearly Physical Exams

Regular check-ups help detect risk factors early and can prevent the progression of conditions like heart disease or diabetes.

Adopting a Heart-Healthy Diet

Consuming foods rich in vegetables, whole grains, lean proteins, and healthy fats while reducing salt and processed food helps maintain heart health.

Regular Exercise

Physical activity like walking, cycling, or swimming strengthens the heart, helps manage weight, and reduces the risk of cardiovascular diseases.

Avoiding Harmful Habits

Avoiding smoking, limiting alcohol consumption, and steering clear of illicit drugs are vital in reducing the risk of developing conditions like heart disease.

Monitoring Blood Pressure and Blood Sugar

Keeping track of these metrics helps identify warning signs early, especially if there is a history of hypertension or diabetes in the family.

For the Black community, where chronic health disparities are more pronounced, knowing and documenting family health history becomes even more vital. Many chronic conditions like hypertension, diabetes, and cancer disproportionately affect Black individuals, and having this information can inform the necessary lifestyle changes and health decisions.

Preventing disease is not just about catching it early when it is easier to manage or treat. Family health history is an invaluable guide that can help steer healthcare decisions and promote better health outcomes for future generations.

Encouraging Family Members to Share

Encouraging open discussions about family health history is essential for creating a proactive approach to disease prevention. For many families, particularly in the Black community, conversations around health can be difficult. There is often a cultural reluctance to speak about medical conditions, especially those that are stigmatized or perceived as weaknesses. However, fostering an environment where family members feel comfortable sharing their health experiences is crucial in closing the gap on preventable diseases.

The first step in encouraging family members to share health information is to create a safe and open space for dialogue. It is crucial to frame the conversation to emphasize the value of this information—not as a critique of past health decisions but as a tool for making informed choices in the future. One way to approach this is by explaining that sharing health information can protect younger generations by providing them with the knowledge needed to anticipate potential health issues and take preventive measures.

For families with older members who may have experienced chronic conditions, it is imperative to collect detailed information. Elders may hold valuable insights about conditions that younger family members may not be aware of, such as the age of onset of certain diseases, complications during treatment, or any genetic predispositions.

To effectively encourage family members to share and document their health information, consider the following strategies:

Create a Comfortable Environment

Choose a comfortable setting where family members feel safe to share their health information. Family gatherings, such as reunions or holidays, can provide an opportunity to start these conversations. Alternatively, consider one-on-one discussions with individual family members to make them feel more at ease.

Start with a Conversation

Begin by initiating a dialogue about the importance of understanding family health history. Approach the topic with sensitivity, recognizing that some family members may be reluctant to discuss health issues due to cultural beliefs, fear, or past experiences with healthcare. Explain how this information can help the family take proactive steps toward better health.

Lead by Example

Share your health information first. Being open about your health history sets the tone for others to follow. Please discuss any health issues you have faced, how you have managed them, and the importance of this information for the family's well-being.

Engage Elders

Encourage older family members to share their health experiences, especially since they often hold the most knowledge about family history. Document their experiences and ask them to recall the health conditions of relatives from previous generations.

Address Concerns about Privacy

Some family members may be concerned about the privacy of their health information. Reassure them that the information will be handled confidentially and only shared with those needing it. Emphasize that the primary goal is to protect and improve the family's health.

Highlight the Benefits

Emphasize the tangible benefits of sharing health information, such as taking preventive measures, catching diseases early, and improving the chances of successful treatment. Explain how this proactive approach can lead to better health outcomes for everyone in the family.

Use Technology to Facilitate Sharing

Encourage using digital tools, such as health apps or online family health history tools, to document and share information. These tools can help organize health data, track trends, and easily share it with healthcare providers. Consider using paper forms or simple questionnaires for family members who are not tech-savvy.

Document and Update Regularly

Encourage family members to document and update their health history regularly as new information becomes available. This ensures that the information remains current and relevant, providing a reliable resource for future generations.

Document Health Information

When documenting family health history, having an organized system is essential for ensuring that critical information is captured accurately. In a previous section, I introduced a structured template to help you gather and record this information efficiently. This template lets you list family members, their ages, known medical conditions, and key health events such as surgeries or major illnesses.

By using this format, you can maintain a clear and accessible record that will be invaluable for both immediate and future reference. This helps you anticipate potential health risks and empowers healthcare providers to offer personalized care based on your family's medical background. I encourage you to revisit this template and use it to support informed decision-making and proactive health management for your family.

Conclusion: Start Now, Secure Tomorrow

Researching our family's health history is not just an exercise in gathering information—it is an investment in your and your family's future. Based on that knowledge, the choices you make today have the power to protect your loved ones from preventable diseases and guide your health journey with clarity and foresight.

It is time to take ownership of your health by actively seeking this crucial information, engaging your family in meaningful conversations, and documenting it thoroughly. These conversations may not always be easy, but they are necessary. By knowing your family's health patterns, you are better equipped to make informed decisions about diet, lifestyle, and medical care that can dramatically influence the quality of life for generations to come.

Remember, acting is not a one-time effort but an ongoing commitment. Start by collecting what you can, encouraging your family members to do the same, and taking steps toward proactive care. Do not wait for a health crisis to prompt these conversations. Empower yourself and your family with knowledge today and use that knowledge to build a healthier future together.

In the Black community, where gaps in health often run deep, we must be even more diligent. Being aware of your family's history is not just about protecting yourself it is about taking collective responsibility for the well-being of your loved ones. Let this chapter serve as the spark that ignites your commitment to acting. Let us honor our health by making family history a part of the foundation we build for better outcomes, more vigorous health, and longer lives. Start today for yourself and your family.

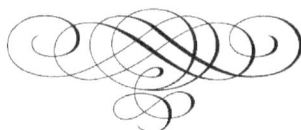

CHAPTER THIRTEEN

COMMUNITY HEALTH INITIATIVES

"True health is built when individuals, families, and communities unite to take action, advocate for change, and support one another on the path to wellness."

THE HEALTH AND WELL-BEING of the Black community are not only shaped by individual actions but by the collective effort of the community at large. Community health initiatives promote wellness, address health disparities, and create lasting change. These programs offer the opportunity to unite individuals, families, and organizations to pursue shared goals whether through educational workshops, health screenings, or advocacy for better healthcare policies. According to the CDC, community health services can support individuals with chronic diseases and help them get the necessary health services by breaking down barriers to care related to social determinants of health.

By coming together, we strengthen our collective power to improve health outcomes for all. In this chapter, we will explore the role of community health programs, how to get involved, and the importance of building partnerships to support community health. It is time to recognize that when we work together, the impact on our health can be profound and far-reaching.

Role of Community Health Programs in Promoting Wellness

Community health programs serve as the foundation for creating healthier communities. These initiatives are often designed to address the specific needs of marginalized groups, including the Black community, who face unique health challenges due to social, economic, and systemic disparities. Programs that promote wellness focus on preventive care, health education, and accessible healthcare services, all of which help reduce the prevalence of chronic diseases and improve overall health outcomes.

For instance, free health screenings and educational workshops on managing chronic diseases like hypertension and diabetes can empower individuals to take control of their health. Additionally, fitness challenges or nutritional education classes can motivate people to make healthier choices. Community health programs also offer vital resources for mental health support, stress management, and building social connections, all essential for well-being.

As a nurse, I cannot underestimate the importance of community health programs in promoting wellness. As inpatient nurses, we discharge many of our patients, especially those with chronic health issues, to follow up with community services to continue care and promote healthy lives, especially among the vulnerable population. One program in California, USA, known as "The Whole Person Care," coordinates care to promote quality healthcare services in communities for better outcomes. This program helps in reaching out to individuals in the community to ensure that they are following up with the medical regimen and assist them with other community services to live a healthier life, such as housing support, transportation, provision of medical supplies, assist with prescription refills and, help remind them of follow up appointments with Primary care doctors.

I believe countries in Africa, like Cameroon, should adopt community health services to promote quality health care to the public, especially to their vulnerable population. Growing up, I had never heard of community health programs designed to meet the healthcare needs of the most susceptible population suffering from long-term diseases. Every healthcare system, including the government hospital, is profit-making (money comes before treatment, unlike in most developed worlds, where treatment comes before payment). A strong and healthy community is a prosperous community.

Examples of Successful Initiatives

A successful example of such an initiative is the "Sister to Sister" program, which focuses on heart health education for Black women. This program has been instrumental in raising awareness about cardiovascular diseases, offering free screenings, and supporting lifestyle changes that reduce the risk of heart disease.

Programs like these demonstrate the critical role community health initiatives play in improving the lives of individuals and families by engaging communities directly and tailoring initiatives to meet their unique needs. Additionally, many other health programs immensely benefit the Black community. Information about these programs and how members of the Black community can continue to benefit from them is provided below.

1. The Black Women's Health Imperative (BWHI)

The Black Women's Health Imperative promotes health equity for Black women and girls. Their programs focus on reducing the incidence of chronic diseases like diabetes, cancer, and heart disease while also promoting reproductive health, mental wellness, and healthy aging. The BWHI provides educational resources, advocacy, and workshops that empower Black women to make informed health decisions.

How the Black Community Can Benefit:

By participating in BWHI programs, Black women can access culturally relevant health education, support groups, and leadership training, helping them manage their health, advocate for their communities, and spread awareness on crucial health issues affecting Black women.

2. REACH (Racial and Ethnic Approaches to Community Health)

REACH is a CDC program designed to reduce racial and ethnic health disparities. It focuses on chronic disease prevention, improving nutrition and physical activity, and reducing tobacco use in underserved communities, including the Black community. REACH programs have been implemented in several cities and counties across the U.S., where they work with local communities to improve access to healthy foods, create safe environments for physical activity, and provide educational resources about chronic disease prevention.

How the Black Community Can Benefit:

The Black community can benefit by engaging in local REACH initiatives and gaining access to community gardens, affordable healthy foods, and complimentary fitness programs. Additionally, these programs create opportunities for health screenings and education about disease prevention.

3. FRESHFARM FoodPrints

FRESHFARM FoodPrints is a school-based program that teaches children in low-income, predominantly Black communities about nutrition, gardening, and cooking healthy meals. The program partners with public schools to provide hands-on lessons, incorporating fresh food from school gardens into meals and promoting lifelong healthy eating habits.

How the Black Community Can Benefit:

Black families can benefit from this program by learning about nutrition and gardening and engaging in healthier eating practices. It fosters an understanding of how to grow and prepare nutritious meals, which can help prevent diet-related diseases like diabetes and hypertension.

4. Healthy Black Pregnancies Initiative (HBPI)

The Healthy Black Pregnancies Initiative aims to reduce the high rates of maternal mortality among Black women. It focuses on prenatal care, education, and support for expecting Black mothers, providing resources to ensure healthy pregnancies and childbirths. The initiative also advocates for better healthcare policies and practices in maternal care to address systemic inequalities. Like many others, it is like Black Infant Health, a program I benefited from a few years ago.

How the Black Community Can Benefit:

Black mothers and families can benefit from prenatal education, access to resources like doulas and midwives, and support networks that promote healthy pregnancy outcomes. This initiative helps ensure that Black mothers receive culturally competent care during their pregnancies, reducing complications and deaths related to childbirth.

5. Anxiety and Depression Association of America (ADAA)

Mental health disorder is one thing that Black people do not talk about easily. Knowledge is lacking, and individuals find seeking help and getting timely support challenging. ADAA is one of the many programs out there supporting Black people with mental health challenges to get the appropriate care they need to understand and overcome mental health issues.

How the Black Community can Benefit:

The Black community can benefit from education on mental health and stigmatization. Understand how to manage issues with anxiety and depression that may be challenging to manage among Black people with all the problems already affecting the Black community, like socio-economic factors and health inequity. They benefit from each other's stories of triumph and tribulation with mental health crises.

6. The Men's Health Network (MHN)

The Men's Health Network is a national organization offering resources and support for addressing men's health issues. The organization focuses on prevention and early detection and conducts screenings and educational campaigns on heart disease, diabetes, cancer, and other chronic diseases.

How the Black Community Can Benefit:

Through MHN, Black men can participate in health screenings, workshops, and outreach programs specifically designed to address chronic illnesses that disproportionately affect them. This program also encourages the early detection of diseases, empowering Black men to seek preventive care and manage their health effectively.

7. The "Whole Person Care" initiative

The "Whole Person Care" initiative is a comprehensive program in California designed to address the needs of vulnerable populations, particularly those with chronic health conditions. This program goes beyond traditional healthcare by focusing on a holistic approach, addressing medical needs and social determinants of health, such as housing, food security, and mental health services. The initiative brings together health services, social services, and community-based organizations to coordinate care for individuals facing complex health challenges.

How the Black Community Can Benefit:

For the Black community, this program offers an invaluable opportunity to receive comprehensive care that considers the broader factors impacting health. By participating in "Whole Person Care," individuals can access resources that help manage chronic diseases like hypertension, diabetes, and heart disease while also receiving support for mental health, housing stability, and other essential services.

The holistic nature of this initiative ensures that members of the Black community are not only treated for their physical ailments but are also supported in ways that promote long-term well-being and resilience. Through such initiatives, the community can take significant strides in closing health disparities and improving overall quality of life.

These programs and several others not mentioned above show how community health initiatives can directly target the unique needs of the Black community, promoting wellness and reducing health disparities. By getting involved, individuals can access the resources and support needed to make informed health decisions, leading to better health outcomes for themselves and their families.

How To Get Involved in Community Health Efforts.

Getting involved in community health efforts is one of the most effective ways to contribute to the well-being of the Black community. These efforts improve individual health outcomes and foster collective action toward reducing health disparities. Whether through volunteering, organizing, or simply participating, every contribution plays a role in building a healthier, more resilient community.

✴ Find a Local Community Health Initiative

The first step in getting involved is finding local community health initiatives that align with your values and needs. Many organizations host health fairs, offer free screenings, and provide workshops welcoming community involvement. Volunteering at these events allows you to contribute time and resources while learning more about your health.

Local hospitals, clinics, and health departments often run programs aimed at addressing chronic health conditions that disproportionately affect the Black community, such as diabetes, hypertension, and asthma. By volunteering, you help others and build connections with healthcare professionals and organizations that can serve as resources for your health journey.

✳ Advocate

Advocacy is another powerful way to get involved. Joining a local health advocacy group, participating in community health forums, or starting conversations about health within your social circles can amplify awareness and drive change. Advocating for better health resources, more accessible healthcare, and culturally competent care are essential steps in closing the gap in health disparities. By raising your voice and mobilizing others, you can help influence policy changes that improve health outcomes for the Black community.

✳ Volunteer

Volunteering is a powerful way to get involved in community health initiatives and make a meaningful impact. By offering your time and skills in local health clinics, you can assist in providing essential care to those in need, particularly within underserved populations. Volunteering to support health literacy programs is another valuable contribution, as it helps individuals understand critical health information, empowering them to make informed decisions about their well-being. You can also help organize health fairs in your community, where residents can receive free health screenings, vaccinations, and educational resources.

These events raise awareness about common health issues, such as hypertension and diabetes, and provide preventive care services that might otherwise be inaccessible. Additionally, offering nutrition programs that promote healthy eating habits is a proactive way to address diet-related diseases.

When you Educate families on balanced diets and healthy food choices, you contribute to reducing the prevalence of obesity, heart disease, and other chronic conditions in the Black community. Volunteering in these areas strengthens individuals' health and fosters a sense of community responsibility, encouraging others to join in creating a healthier, more informed population.

Practical Ways to Get Involved

Many successful programs have shown how grassroots involvement can drive meaningful change, but there is always room for more hands and voices in the mission to close health disparities. Here is how you can get involved today.

Advocacy for Health Policies

Engaging with local leaders and policymakers to push for policies that ensure equitable healthcare for the Black community is essential. Whether speaking out at town halls or working with advocacy groups, every voice can make a difference in demanding better resources for underrepresented populations. Pushing for increased funding for local health centers or advocating for laws that provide easier access to preventive care is a step forward in ensuring health equity.

Support Groups and Peer Counseling

Joining or initiating peer support groups can foster community while addressing health concerns. These groups provide spaces for shared experiences, emotional support, and practical advice. By creating or becoming part of these networks, individuals can contribute to a supportive environment where health is prioritized and collective efforts promote well-being.

Fundraising for Health Programs

Supporting local health programs does not always require medical expertise. Organizing or participating in fundraisers can have a lasting impact by providing financial support to health outreach efforts, free screenings, and wellness workshops. These resources are often crucial in reaching more people and delivering unavailable essential services.

Health Ambassador Programs

Many cities offer health ambassador programs, where community members receive training to educate others about important health issues. Becoming a health ambassador allows individuals to lead within their communities by spreading awareness of disease prevention, nutrition, and available health services. It is an impactful way to ensure that health education reaches every corner of our communities.

Partnering with Faith-Based Organizations

Churches and faith-based groups have always been central to the Black community. By working with these organizations, we can expand health outreach efforts and create programs that address physical and spiritual wellness. Hosting fitness activities, health talks, or screenings through faith-based groups can build trust and reach individuals without access to other healthcare support.

The pathway to better health of the Black community does not solely rest in the hands of medical professionals it lies within all of us. When we step up, get involved, and encourage others to join us, we become the change-makers in our communities. The examples we have shared, from volunteering to advocacy, demonstrate the wide range of opportunities available to those looking to make an impact. It is not just about receiving healthcare but about actively contributing to it, advocating for it, and ensuring that our Black community benefits fully from the resources and knowledge available.

Getting involved does not always require significant commitments of time or resources. Even small steps, such as sharing health information with friends and family or encouraging others to attend local health events, can significantly impact the situation. These seemingly small actions can ripple out and make a big difference. The more people in our community who are informed and engaged in their health, the stronger and healthier our collective future becomes.

Building Partnerships to Support Community Health

Creating a healthier community is a shared responsibility that cannot be achieved by individuals or health organizations alone. It requires the collective efforts of different stakeholders healthcare providers, community leaders, educators, local businesses, and faith-based organizations all coming together to address the unique health needs of the Black community. Your collaboration is not just important; it's crucial. Partnerships are critical in bridging the gaps within our healthcare system, particularly for underserved populations.

Building effective partnerships in community health ensures that resources are maximized, and outreach efforts are extended to those who need them the most. When local organizations collaborate with healthcare institutions, for instance, they can create more accessible and sustainable programs that cater to the specific health challenges faced by the Black community, such as diabetes, hypertension, and mental health issues. Additionally, partnerships help to bring a diversity of expertise and resources, which enriches the impact of community health initiatives.

The key to building solid partnerships lies in understanding the shared goals and the unique contributions each partner can bring. For example, healthcare providers may offer medical services and screenings, while local businesses or faith-based organizations can provide space for health workshops or educational sessions. Educators can help by promoting health literacy and creating awareness campaigns that address preventive care and lifestyle changes.

Examples of Successful Partnerships

One notable example of successful partnership-building is the collaboration between community health centers and local schools in offering wellness programs. These programs focus on providing students and their families access to preventive care, vaccinations, and health education, all within the school setting. Such partnerships address students' health needs and encourage parents and guardians to implement preventive healthcare practices.

Another example is the partnership between national health organizations and Black-owned businesses. Through initiatives like free health screenings at community events or sponsored fitness programs, these partnerships promote awareness and encourage individuals to take charge of their health in familiar, trusted environments. These partnerships have been instrumental in normalizing conversations around health in the Black community and ensuring that care reaches those who may not frequent traditional healthcare settings.

Steps to Building Partnerships

Starting with a shared vision is essential to building partnerships that support community health successfully. Bringing together stakeholders who share a common goal such as reducing health disparities or increasing access to preventive care ensures everyone is working toward the same outcome. Open communication is critical to maintaining strong partnerships, allowing for regular updates, feedback, and adjustments to strategies as needed.

Likewise, leveraging existing community networks is an effective way to create trusting partnerships. Faith-based organizations, local businesses, and schools are all deeply ingrained in the fabric of the Black community, making them ideal partners for health initiatives. These entities can serve as entry points to the community, helping health professionals reach people who may otherwise feel disconnected from the healthcare system.

Another critical factor is sustainability. For a partnership to have a long-lasting impact, it must be nurtured and maintained over time. Regular evaluations of progress and outcomes can help identify areas for improvement and ensure that the partnership continues to serve its intended purpose. Community health partnerships can evolve and grow by fostering long-term relationships and continually adapting to the population's changing needs.

Benefits of Partnerships for the Black Community

For the Black community, these partnerships provide numerous benefits. They improve access to healthcare, raise awareness about preventable diseases, and create opportunities for individuals to participate in their healthcare journey. We can build a healthier, more resilient community that prioritizes prevention, health education, and overall well-being by working together. These partnerships serve as a bridge to overcome systemic barriers, ensuring everyone has the resources and support they need to live healthier lives.

Realizing that we are interrelated as a community is essential. Building partnerships among private and public healthcare systems is one way to promote quality healthcare. Individuals should be able to access the closest clinic or emergency department without fearing high hospital costs or billing. Hospitals building partnerships with pharmacies, hospitals building partnerships with social services, or pharmacies building partnerships with insurance companies may quickly help community members get the right healthcare services on time.

Hospitals can partner with homeless shelters so that patients suffering from homelessness with chronic health issues are not sent back onto the street. It is difficult to manage certain chronic health conditions on the street, especially not knowing where to store medications. Partnership is essential to reduce healthcare burden and promote quality and better outcomes.

Advocating for Better Health Resources and Policies in Your Community.

Advocacy is a powerful tool for driving change in healthcare systems and ensuring that the needs of the Black community are not overlooked. While individual actions such as adopting healthier lifestyles and engaging in preventive care are critical, systemic changes are necessary to address the health disparities that disproportionately affect Black individuals. Advocacy works to influence public health policies, increase access to healthcare resources, and bring the reforms needed to create a more equitable healthcare environment.

To advocate effectively for better health resources, individual members and community leaders must first understand their communities' specific needs and challenges. This involves identifying gaps in access to care, education, and health services and then working to address these gaps through collective action. For example, many Black communities face a shortage of healthcare providers, lack access to affordable care, or struggle with implicit bias within healthcare settings. Advocates can push for changes that improve health outcomes by raising awareness of these issues.

One cannot underestimate the importance of advocacy in health care. Advocacy is needed to make significant changes that benefit the community, especially in health care, where the people who need help are already in vulnerable states.

One reason I'm writing this book, *My Health, My Priority*, is because I believe the black population still needs more voices to advocate on their behalf to implement healthcare reforms targeting Africans, granting them more access to health care, promoting health literacy in the African community, and including diversified healthcare workforce to meet the socio-economic and health care need of the African people that are already affected by chronic health challenges.

Seeing all these young Africans with health issues like heart failure, diabetes, and hypertension and reading all these studies with data analyzing the prevalence of chronic diseases among Africans as compared is a concern and a call for advocacy for health services targeting the Black population. The question is, how many Black people participate in policymaking affecting black health? I believe that inclusivity and diversity should be present in every department of the healthcare system. One can improve healthcare practices by advocating for the right course of action.

Steps to Advocate for Better Health Resources

1. Raise Awareness

The first step in advocacy is raising awareness about the Black community's health disparities. This can be done through community meetings, social media campaigns, and educational workshops highlighting specific challenges, such as higher rates of chronic diseases, limited access to quality care, or the effects of socioeconomic factors on health. Engaging local media and community leaders in these conversations can help amplify the message and reach a broader audience.

2. Get Involved in Policy Discussions

Advocacy goes beyond awareness it also involves actively participating in policy discussions at the local, state, and national levels. Attend town hall meetings, write to local representatives, and collaborate with organizations that work on public health policy. Pushing for policies that improve healthcare access, such as Medicaid expansion or funding for community health programs, can have a lasting impact on the health of the Black community.

3. Support Health Education Initiatives

One of the most effective ways to advocate for better health resources is to support and promote health education initiatives within the community. These could include workshops on preventive care, managing chronic illnesses, or understanding family health history. Health education empowers individuals to make informed decisions about their health and encourages them to seek the necessary resources.

4. Partner with Advocacy Organizations

There are several advocacy organizations focused on improving health equity in Black communities. Partnering with groups such as the National Medical Association, the Black Women's Health Imperative, or local health coalitions can provide a platform for your advocacy efforts. These organizations often have the resources, networks, and expertise needed to effect real change, and working with them can amplify the voices of those in your community.

Challenges in Advocacy

Advocating for better health resources is not without its challenges. Systemic barriers such as racism, economic inequality, and political resistance can make it challenging to achieve the desired changes. Additionally, there may be a lack of engagement or trust within the community due to historical mistreatment in healthcare settings. Overcoming these challenges requires persistence, collaboration, and a clear understanding of the community's needs.

Building trust is essential in advocacy work. Creating spaces where community members feel heard, and their concerns are taken seriously is necessary. Being transparent about goals and strategies and involving community leaders in decision-making can help build the trust needed for successful advocacy.

The Impact of Successful Advocacy

Advocacy for better health resources has already significantly impacted various communities nationwide. These efforts have shown that change is possible when people come together for a common cause, from increasing funding for community health centers to advocating for policies that reduce health disparities.

For example, successful advocacy campaigns have led to expanded access to Medicaid, which has provided millions of low-income individuals, including many in the Black community, with access to affordable healthcare. Other campaigns have focused on improving maternal health outcomes for Black women, addressing mental health disparities, or increasing access to vaccinations and screenings in underserved areas.

As we continue to advocate for better health resources and policies, we must remain committed to improving healthcare access, reducing disparities, and ensuring that every member of the Black community can lead a healthy, fulfilling life. We can drive meaningful change in the healthcare system by raising awareness, participating in policy discussions, and supporting health education initiatives.

The power of advocacy lies in collective action; together, we can create the equitable healthcare environment that our community deserves. Let us take the steps needed to advocate for better health policies, ensuring our families, friends, and neighbors have the necessary resources to thrive.

Conclusion: Choose to Build Healthier Black Communities Together with Us

As we close this chapter, it is essential to reflect on the power we hold in transforming the health outcomes of our communities. This transformation begins with each of us but cannot end there it must ripple outward, reaching our families, neighbors, and the larger Black community. We have explored the significance of family health history, community involvement, and advocacy for health policies, but now it is time to implement those lessons.

The road ahead is a collective effort. Begin by taking charge of your health and using the tools and resources available to make informed decisions. Then, extend knowledge to your family by encouraging them to document their health histories and make healthier choices. Become actively involved in community health initiatives by volunteering, organizing health fairs, or simply sharing your newfound knowledge with others.

As members of the Black community, our individual actions may seem insignificant, but together, they form a powerful force for change. By forging partnerships, advocating for better policies, and committing to the health of others, we can strengthen the entire community. This is not just a personal journey—it's a shared mission for all of us to rise, educate, and empower, and it's through our collective action that we can make a real difference.

The steps you take today can shape a healthier, more equitable future for future generations. Embrace this responsibility, knowing that your actions not only improve your health but also contribute to a stronger, more resilient community. Your role in this mission is crucial, and your actions can make a real difference.

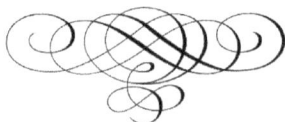

CHAPTER FOURTEEN

YOUR HEALTH YOUR PRIORITY

"When you prioritize your health, you shape a better future for yourself, your family, and the Black and African Community."

IN THIS BOOK, WE have delved deeply into the most pressing health issues affecting the Black community. From understanding the systemic barriers in Part One, which highlights the disparities in healthcare access, to exploring preventive measures in Part Two, we have equipped ourselves with knowledge on how to take proactive steps toward better health. Throughout Part Three, we took a closer look at disease-specific management, emphasizing the importance of taking charge of our well-being.

However, at the heart of it all is one undeniable truth: your health is your responsibility. The Black community faces numerous challenges, including higher rates of chronic diseases and limited access to healthcare resources, but true empowerment begins when everyone takes ownership of their well-being. As we have seen in previous chapters, relying on external systems or hoping someone else will prioritize our health is not enough. This chapter, like the book, is about encouraging you to act.

When you understand your family health history, embrace healthy lifestyle choices, and leverage community resources, you can take practical steps to ensure your health remains a priority. It is time to turn the insights from this book into daily habits, recognizing that health is more than the absence of illness it is the pursuit of wellness for us, our families, and our community. Let us work together to make *My Health, My Priority* a reality for each of us.

Understanding the Importance of Taking Charge

Knowing that you are in control of your health and not the health professionals is essential. Remember the saying, "The patients are always right." As an individual, you have power over your health and oversee the decision-making of your health care. If you manage your health, you may reduce the number of times you see a doctor or a nurse; you may reduce the need for medical management unless necessary. That is because you oversee your health.

Taking charge of your health is particularly vital for the Black community, where genetic predisposition, systemic inequalities, and cultural factors often contribute to higher rates of chronic illnesses. Taking proactive steps toward managing your health reduces your risk of developing preventable diseases and breaks the cycle of health disparities that disproportionately affect our community.

When we actively engage in our well-being whether through balanced nutrition, regular exercise, or mental health care we build resilience against conditions prevalent in the Black community, such as hypertension, diabetes, and heart disease. Taking charge means not waiting for illness to strike but staying informed and making daily decisions that prioritize health. It is about knowing our family health history, recognizing early warning signs, and advocating for the care we need.

For the African and Black diaspora, where access to quality healthcare may be limited or delayed, being in control of our health empowers us to make informed decisions and seek timely medical attention. It also ensures we pass on healthier habits and knowledge to the next generation, creating a legacy of wellness that counteracts the systemic barriers we have faced. Taking charge of our health means we are not just surviving we are thriving, ensuring that we live longer, healthier lives for ourselves, our families, and our communities.

Your health is your responsibility; making positive changes is never too late. By prioritizing your health, you can prevent chronic diseases, manage existing conditions, and improve your quality of life. This chapter focuses on practical strategies to help you take control of your health. Remember, prioritizing your well-being is not a selfish act; it benefits those around you, particularly in the Black community, where health disparities continue to affect many.

Priority Points:

✶ Having Your Family Health Knowledge Is Powerful

As discussed in *Chapter Ten*, understanding your family health history is one of the most powerful tools for taking control of your health. By knowing your risks, you can be proactive and make informed decisions to safeguard your well-being.

✶ Embrace Preventive Care

In *Chapter Three*, we emphasized the value of preventive care. Making regular appointments for check-ups and screenings is one of the simplest ways to take charge of your health and prevent minor issues from becoming primary concerns.

✶ Cultivate a Healthy Lifestyle for a Healthier Future

In *Chapter Four*, we explored the importance of adopting a healthy lifestyle. The everyday decisions—like eating a balanced diet and staying active—give you the power to shape your health for the better.

✴ Leverage Community Health Resources

In *Chapter Eleven*, we saw how community health programs are a crucial resource can be. Taking charge of your health does not mean you must do it alone. There are programs and networks to support you every step of the way.

✴ Always Advocate for Your Health

Throughout the book, particularly in *Chapter Six* and *Chapter Eleven*, we have talked about the importance of advocating for yourself in healthcare settings. Do not be afraid to ask questions, seek second opinions, and ensure you receive the care you deserve.

Implementing Healthy Habits

Taking charge of your health means implementing healthy habits. Your health is fragile like an eggshell; you must guard it by intentionally making healthy habits. Drink more water instead of soda and alcohol; eat more vegetables and whole grains instead of white rice; and be active instead of passive.

Associate with trusted individuals who uplift your spirit and promote a sense of belonging. Take prescription drugs instead of self-medications. Stop smoking. Remember that your habits can determine the course of your health in disease prevention and health maintenance. For example, an individual with type 2 diabetes can manage it with a lifestyle without any medical regimen.

Building and maintaining healthy habits is about personal discipline and creating a lifestyle that aligns with our goals and values. Implementing these habits requires intentionality and a focus on sustainability, ensuring that our changes fit seamlessly into our daily lives.

One critical approach to implementing healthy habits is setting clear, achievable goals. When we aim for significant lifestyle changes all at once, the process can become overwhelming and unsustainable. We can gradually introduce healthier choices into our routines by starting with small, measurable goals. For example, rather than aiming for an hour of exercise each day, beginning with 10 or 15 minutes of physical activity can provide a manageable start that builds momentum over time.

Another important aspect of habit formation is understanding our triggers and routines. Often, unhealthy habits are ingrained because they are part of a routine, such as reaching for snacks while watching TV or skipping meals due to a busy schedule. By recognizing these patterns, we can intentionally shift our routines to support healthier behaviors. This could mean preparing healthy snacks ahead of time or scheduling regular mealtimes, ensuring we nourish our bodies properly throughout the day.

Accountability is another powerful tool for implementing healthy habits. Sharing our goals with others whether through support groups, friends, or family creates a sense of commitment and provides external motivation. Having someone to check in with or participate in a healthy habit strengthens the resolve to stick to it. Additionally, joining wellness communities or participating in group fitness activities can create a sense of belonging and encouragement, which makes the journey towards better health more enjoyable.

Healthy habits also require self-compassion and flexibility. There will inevitably be setbacks, days when we miss our exercise or indulge in less nutritious food options. Instead of seeing these moments as failures, it is essential to view them as part of the process and allow us the grace to start fresh the next day. What matters most is the consistency and long-term commitment to making better choices, not the occasional slip-ups.

Lastly, integrating healthy habits into a broader purpose can create deeper motivation. When we see our health as part of a larger vision whether it is staying active to spend more time with loved ones, improving mental well-being for career growth, or maintaining physical vitality to give back to our communities it becomes easier to prioritize health in our daily lives.

Priority Points:

★ Start Small, Stay Consistent

In Chapter Four, we learned that adopting a healthy lifestyle is not about making drastic changes overnight but instead about consistently incorporating small, manageable habits that accumulate over time. Begin with small steps, such as adding more fruit and vegetables to your meals or taking 10-15 minutes daily for light physical activity. Consistency is critical to long-term success as these small efforts grow into solid, sustainable routines.

✴ Establishing a Routine

As discussed in *Chapter Five*, managing stress and mental health is integral to overall well-being. Create a daily routine that includes time for relaxation, mindfulness practices, and stress-relieving exercises like walking, stretching, or meditation. Implementing a regular sleep schedule can also dramatically impact both your mental and physical health.

✴ Utilizing Available Resources

In *Chapter Eleven*, we touched on the importance of community health resources. Whether joining a local fitness class, accessing a nutritionist, or participating in community health screenings, use what is available in your community to support your new healthy habits. These programs can serve as a support system and provide guidance, accountability, and motivation.

Incorporate Physical Activity into Daily Life

In Chapter Four, we discussed the benefits of regular exercise. Simple ways to integrate physical activity include walking instead of driving short distances, taking the stairs rather than the elevator, and finding a form of exercise you enjoy, such as dancing, yoga, or sports. Regular movement helps manage weight, reduce stress, and strengthen the heart.

Make Mindful Choices About Food

Chapter Four highlights that a balanced diet is crucial to maintaining good health. Focus on eating whole, nutrient-dense foods such as vegetables, fruits, whole grains, lean proteins, and healthy fats. Avoid processed foods and sugary drinks. Building a mindful approach to eating ensures you nourish your body while preventing common chronic conditions like diabetes and heart disease.

Leveraging Community Resources

Leveraging community resources is a powerful strategy for improving overall well-being in the Black community. Resources such as local health programs, faith-based initiatives, and wellness networks can support individuals seeking to maintain or improve their health.

These resources often provide access to free or low-cost services, including health screenings, educational workshops, fitness programs, and nutrition counseling. For individuals who may not have access to private healthcare or comprehensive insurance, community health centers offer invaluable services that address preventive care and chronic disease management. By utilizing these resources, members of the Black community can take proactive steps toward better health, regardless of financial or social barriers.

Faith-based organizations play a particularly significant role in the Black community. Churches and other religious institutions often serve as health education and outreach hubs, organizing events such as health fairs, vaccination drives, and mental health workshops. These initiatives provide essential health services and foster community and trust, encouraging individuals to prioritize their health in a supportive environment.

Additionally, social and support groups within the community can be vital for sharing information, building accountability, and encouraging one another on health journeys. Whether it is a local fitness group, a diabetes support network, or an online platform focused on health literacy, these spaces create a collective effort toward wellness. By joining such groups, individuals can benefit from shared experiences, peer guidance, and motivation, all of which contribute to long-term health improvements.

Accessing community resources also extends to partnering with local organizations and advocates fighting health equity. These partnerships can offer more comprehensive support, from helping individuals navigate the healthcare system to advocating for better health policies directly impacting the Black community. Being part of a more significant movement toward health equality empowers individuals to improve their health and contribute to systemic change.

Leveraging the knowledge in *My Health, My Priority* is also essential, as the Black community must navigate the unique challenges they face concerning health disparities. This book provides tailored insights and strategies that address the specific health issues prevalent within the community, such as cardiovascular diseases, diabetes, and access to preventive care.

Offering practical advice on how to take charge of one's health, this book serves as a vital tool for individuals looking to improve their well-being through informed decision-making and lifestyle changes. My Health, My Priority, goes beyond individual health, encouraging readers to engage with their families and communities to create a collective wellness approach. It provides the knowledge and empowerment needed to leverage personal habits and community resources effectively, making it an indispensable guide for anyone committed to prioritizing their health.

As you seek to take advantage of all the available health resources in our community, get involved in building the community and strengthening one another. Volunteer for community services, join support groups to offer free food to homeless centers, help organize health fairs, and help with educational services to improve health literacy in the community. Share ideas on available resources in the community to help meet their health needs, involve yourself in discussions that can promote quality of life, and be open to innovative ideas.

Priority Activities

✴ Utilize *My Health, My Priority* book as a Vital Resource

My Health, My Priority is a comprehensive resource for the Black community. It equips individuals with practical tools and knowledge to take charge of their health. Utilizing this book alongside community-based programs ensures a well-rounded approach to wellness.

✴ Understand the Value of Local Health Programs

In *Chapter Eleven*, we discussed the importance of community health programs in promoting wellness. These programs, such as the "Sister to Sister" initiative, provide essential services like screenings and health education tailored explicitly to the Black community's needs.

✴ Prioritize Preventive Care through Accessible Community Resources

As emphasized in *Chapter Three*, preventive care is critical to improving health outcomes. Community resources, like local clinics and wellness programs, offer accessible regular check-ups and early detection opportunities, which are essential in preventing chronic diseases.

✶ Embrace Healthy Habits with Community Support

Chapter Four emphasized the significance of adopting healthy lifestyle habits. Participating in community-based fitness programs or nutrition workshops can provide the guidance and support needed to implement and maintain these habits.

✶ Leverage Community Partnerships for Health Advocacy

Chapter Eleven also explored the role of community partnerships in health advocacy. Leveraging these partnerships can help you navigate complex healthcare systems and push for policies that improve health access and outcomes for the Black community.

✶ Harness the Power of Community Accountability

As discussed throughout the book, the collective power of community support fosters accountability and motivation. Engaging with local wellness networks and support groups can enhance personal commitment to health and provide a shared sense of purpose on the journey to wellness.

Creating a Health Action Plan

Taking charge of your health requires more than just knowledge it calls for actionable steps to reach your wellness goals consistently. A health action plan serves as a roadmap, guiding you through the daily habits, preventive measures, and healthcare practices necessary for maintaining your health and well-being.

Developing a personal health action plan can be transformative for the Black community where health disparities persist. It enables individuals and families to take control of their wellness, prevent chronic conditions, and improve long-term health outcomes.

A health action plan is an intentional, structured approach focusing on clear objectives, regular check-ins, and accountability. This plan addresses your current health concerns and anticipates potential risks, mainly if certain diseases run in your family. By focusing on preventive care, healthy lifestyle choices, and leveraging community resources, you can build a sustainable plan that works for you and supports your overall well-being.

Recognizing how your lifestyle can affect your health, it is time to start taking healthy actions to promote a better quality of life. Developing a realistic action plan to keep you in check is essential. For example, how many days a week will you exercise, and how many hours per exercise? Stay committed to planning.

Here is how to create an effective health action plan:

1. Set Clear Health Goals

Start by identifying the areas of your health that need attention. This might include managing weight, lowering blood pressure, improving mental health, or increasing physical activity. Be specific about what you want to achieve, and make sure your goals are measurable and realistic. For example, if your goal is to lower your blood pressure, set a target range and timeline to achieve it.

2. Prioritize Preventive Care

Ensure your plan includes regular screenings, vaccinations, and check-ups based on your family health history and individual risk factors. Early detection can significantly reduce the risk of complications from chronic diseases like diabetes, hypertension, and cancer. Preventive care should be the backbone of your action plan, supporting your efforts to maintain long-term health.

3. Incorporate Daily Healthy Habits

Include specific habits that support your physical, mental, and emotional well-being. This may involve a balanced diet, regular physical activity, adequate sleep, and stress management techniques. The focus is not just on what you avoid but on what you actively incorporate into your daily life to promote wellness.

4. Utilize Community Resources

As we have explored in earlier chapters, numerous resources are available to support your health journey, from community wellness programs to local clinics offering free or low-cost health services. Make these resources a part of your plan and take advantage of the support they provide.

5. Build Accountability

Whether through family members, friends, or local support groups, accountability is crucial to sticking with your health plan. Share your goals with someone you trust or join a group with similar health objectives. This provides motivation and ensures that you stay on track.

6. Evaluate and Adjust Your Plan

A health action plan is not static. Life and health conditions change, so your plan should be flexible enough to adapt to new challenges. Regularly evaluate your progress and adjust as needed, whether that means increasing your activity levels, reassessing your dietary choices, or scheduling additional healthcare appointments.

Template for Creating a Health Action Plan

It is time to turn every insight this book shares into action. I have carefully designed this health action plan template to empower you to take control of your health in a structured and achievable way. This template will guide you in setting clear health goals, identifying preventive care needs, building healthy daily routines, and staying accountable.

As you fill it out, remember that your health is your priority, and by taking these steps, you are investing in a healthier future for yourself and our Black community. This tool is meant to be adaptable, so feel free to personalize it according to your specific needs and circumstances.

Health Goal	Preventive Care	Daily Habits	Community Resources	Accountability	Evaluation
Example: Lower Blood Pressure	Regular blood pressure monitoring, annual check-ups	Low-sodium diet, 30 minutes of daily exercise, stress management	Join a local hypertension support group	Share progress with a family member or group	Check blood pressure weekly, adjust diet/exercise as needed
Example: Manage Weight	Regular weight check-ins, screenings for related conditions	A balanced diet, limited sugar intake, 45 minutes of exercise	Attend a community fitness class, consult a nutritionist	Work with a partner to stay accountable	Track weight monthly, adjust activity levels as needed
Example: Mental Health Well-being	Annual mental health check-ups, screenings for depression	Practice mindfulness, maintain a consistent sleep schedule	Participate in community-based mental health workshops	Partner with a mental health support group	Monitor mood and stress levels weekly and adjust self-care routines as needed.
Your Health Goal					

This template provides a simple and practical framework for organizing your health priorities and creating a personalized plan. Please share it with a friend so they can stay accountable to each other for consistency.

Conclusion: Your Health, Our Pride

As we reach the end of this chapter and this book, I encourage you to incorporate the knowledge and insights we have explored into your daily life. Your health is your priority, and the power to shape your well-being lies in the decisions you make each day.

This is not just about understanding the importance of preventive care, healthy habits, or community resources—it is about acting, creating a plan, and holding yourself accountable for the steps you take toward better health.

The journey to disease prevention and health maintenance is not one you must take alone. Whether through family, friends, or community health programs, you have the support and resources to help you succeed. Should you have any questions or need guidance as you navigate this path, I am here to support you.

The last pages of this book include my contact information, and I invite you to reach out. Let us work together to ensure that you and the Black community thrive in health, now and for future generations. Your health is our pride—make it count. Remember, you are not alone on this journey. I am here to support you every step of the way.

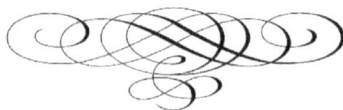

CONCLUSION

AS WE CONCLUDE *My Health, My Priority*, I am grateful for your commitment to better health and well-being. Your journey through this book is a testament to your dedication to yourself and our community. Your commitment is a responsibility, and it has the power to bring about meaningful change. Thank you for being a part of this.

Throughout this book, we have delved into some of the most prevalent chronic health issues that disproportionately affect the Black community. From cardiovascular diseases to metabolic, endocrine disorders, and respiratory diseases, the information shared here is not just knowledge but practical strategies that you can easily integrate into your life. Remember, it's not just about knowing but about applying this knowledge to make a tangible difference in your health.

Envision the positive ripple effects if we take a few steps towards healthier living. Imagine a community where fewer people suffer from preventable diseases, the inflated costs of chronic illnesses do not burden families, and our children grow up with a better understanding of health and wellness. This vision can become a reality, but it starts with each act.

Consider the ways you can integrate the advice from this book into your daily life:

Adopt Healthy Eating Habits: Eat more fruits, vegetables, and whole grains. Reducing salt, sugar, and unhealthy fat intake can significantly lower your risk of many chronic diseases.

Stay Active: Regular physical activity is not just about losing weight it is about keeping your heart healthy, reducing stress, and improving overall well-being. Find an activity you enjoy and make it a routine.

Regular Health Screenings: Early detection is critical in managing many health conditions. Schedule regular check-ups and screenings for hypertension, diabetes, and cancer. This proactive approach can catch potential issues before they become serious.

Community Engagement: Share what you have learned with others. Please encourage your family and friends to prioritize their health. Together, we can create a culture of wellness and support.

Your health is indeed your greatest asset. By prioritizing it, you invest in a brighter, healthier future for yourself and those around you. The determination and conviction you gain from this book are the tools you need to make lasting changes.

Remember, the information and strategies in this book are just the beginning. The fundamental transformation happens when you put these principles into practice. Take the first step today: making a healthier food choice, walking, or scheduling an overdue health check-up. No matter how small, each action is a step towards a healthier you and a stronger community.

I appreciate your dedication to improving your health and being part of this vital movement. Together, we can reduce health disparities, improve lives, and build a future where wellness is within everyone's reach.

Now, let us take the knowledge we have gained and turn it into action through the commitment to a healthy lifestyle below. Our health, our community, and our pride depend on it.

Your Commitment to a Healthy Lifestyle

I, _____, commit to prioritizing my health and well-being. I pledge to make informed choices that support a healthier lifestyle for myself and my community.

I will:

* Embrace nutritious eating habits and incorporate more fruits, vegetables, and whole grains into my diet.

* Engage in regular physical activity to keep my body strong and resilient.

* Schedule and attend regular health screenings to detect and address potential health issues early.

* Prioritize my mental and emotional wellness through mindfulness, seeking support, and nurturing my social connections.

* Share my knowledge and encourage others to take proactive steps towards better health.

By taking these actions, I am investing in a brighter, healthier future for myself and those around me. Together, we can build a community where wellness and vitality are within everyone's reach.

Signature: _____

Date: _____

MOVING FORWARD WITH YOUR COMMITMENT

CONGRATULATIONS ON MAKING this important commitment to your health and well-being. We have designed a comprehensive workbook and training program to help you turn these commitments into lasting habits. This program is tailored to guide you step-by-step through adopting healthier lifestyle choices and overcoming any challenges you may face.

The workbook contains practical exercises, actionable plans, and valuable resources to help you stay on track with your goals. The training program offers additional support, including workshops, expert advice, and a community of like-minded individuals dedicated to improving their health.

Participating in the training program will give you the tools and confidence needed to make sustainable changes, ensuring your commitment to a healthier lifestyle becomes a reality. Together, we can achieve better health outcomes and foster a stronger, more vibrant community.

Please fill out this form and send its photo to miranmiry@yahoo.com with "Free Coaching" In the subject line:

Full Name: _____

Email Address: _____

Home City/Town: _____

WhatsApp Number: _____

Occupation: _____

What help do you need?

_____

_____

_____

_____

_____

_____

Congratulations on joining us on this transformative journey. In return, let us make a lasting impact on your health and our community. Your next step awaits in the training program, where we will provide the tailored guidance and support you need to succeed.

SEE YOU IN CLASS.

ABOUT THE AUTHOR

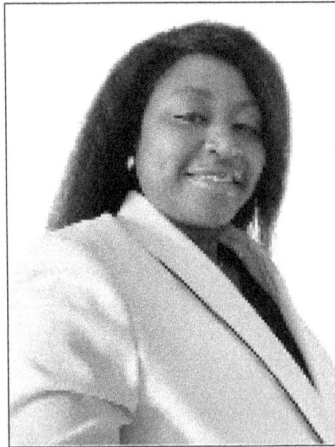

WITH A RICH AND DIVERSE background in clinical nursing, Miranda has dedicated over a decade to the healthcare profession, establishing herself as a passionate advocate for patient care, education, and community health. As a certified Med-Surg Registered Nurse (CMS-RN) and an experienced Clinical Nurse, she has worked extensively in the med-surg/telemetry unit since 2015, where she has proven her expertise in clinical nursing, direct patient care, and leadership as a charge nurse in a fifty-four beds acute care unit. Her commitment to nursing education and mentorship is demonstrated through her role as a preceptor for nursing students and a mentor for new nurses.

In addition to her bedside nursing, she has served on various hospital committees, such as the Fall Committee, unit-based shared governance, and the Code Blue Committee. She has also been a champion of telemetry and Clinical Opioid Withdrawal Assessment (COWS) education. Her hands-on experience and her roles in these leadership and educational capacities have further honed her clinical judgment, adaptability, and passion for equitable healthcare practices.

Since 2023, she has embraced a new chapter in her career as a Clinical Nursing Instructor, where she teaches and guides nursing students in clinical settings. Her commitment to developing future healthcare professionals reflects her dedication to fostering clinical excellence and instilling critical thinking skills in her students. Known for her calm and steady demeanor under pressure, she strongly advocates for fair practices and compassionate care, making her a role model and authority in her field.

In her academic pursuits, Miranda holds a Master of Science in Nursing (MSN) focusing on Nurse Education, further cementing her role as a thought leader in healthcare education.

Beyond her professional accomplishments, she founded the Hope Outreach Program for Education (Hope

Foundation) in 2020. Through this charitable foundation, she offers free back-to-school supplies to students in her local African community, exemplifying her dedication to improving lives beyond the hospital setting.

Her passion for education, justice, and community service extends naturally into her work in this book, *My Health, My Priority*. As an advocate for health literacy in the Black community, she uses her vast experience and compassionate approach to highlight the importance of proactive healthcare, preventive care, and empowering individuals to take charge of their well-being. Her deep-rooted commitment to equitable healthcare makes her a credible and authoritative voice on these vital health issues.

www.ingramcontent.com/pod-product-compliance
Lightning Source LLC
Chambersburg PA
CBHW031426270326
41930CB00007B/594